Sleep, Drugs & Alzheimer's Disease

A book for The
Alzheimers Prevention
Project

By
Larry D. Reid
And
Valerie A. Lavash

Cognitive Behavioral Therapy for Insomnia

"If what we *do* modifies what we *are,* then that opens *the possibility to use behavioral technologies to modify our physiology to become what we wish to be.*"

Stated another way: "Everything is the way it is because it got that way." D'Arcy Thompson

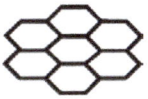

Sleep

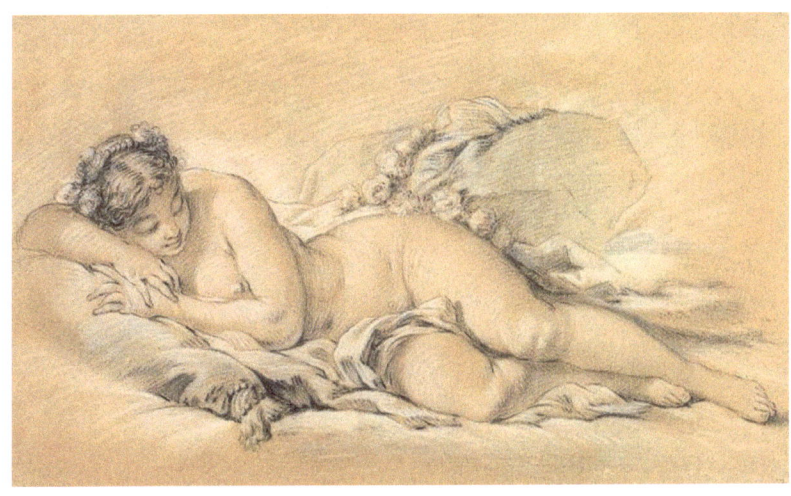

Young Woman Sleeping, c.1760-Francois Boucher-WikiArt.org

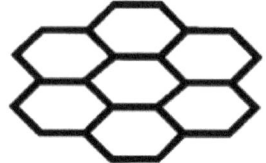

ISBN-13: 9781730889271
ISBN-10: 1730889271

This book is published by Hexagon, Brunswick, NY.

© 2018 Larry D. Reid. All rights reserved. This book was printed by CreateSpace and is available by way of Amazon Books.

Preface

This book was written for those willing to make changes in their daily lives to prevent themselves from developing Alzheimer's disease. Two such changes are to improve one's quality of sleep and avoid certain kinds of drugs.

The Alzheimers Prevention Project is a program of activities designed to engage citizens in activities that will significantly reduce their risk of developing late-onset Alzheimer's disease (LOAD). The staff of the Project has identified poor sleep as one of the main factors that clearly increases the risk of developing LOAD. These risk-factors includes poor diet, lack of physical exercise, lack of certain kinds of cognitive exercise, loss of olfaction and polypharmacy. This book focuses on the risk-factors of insomnia and drugs used to treat insomnia; two factors that seem particularly pertinent to developing LOAD.

The Alzheimers Prevention Project involves faculty and students studying at Rensselaer Polytechnic Institute. The group has been investigating ways to prevent Alzheimer's disease for several years. This scholarly activity resulted in some pilot studies exploring the relationship between disrupted olfactory perception and the development of Alzheimer's disease. Our scholarly activity produced reviews of the literature supporting our ideas about how to prevent LOAD.

As we did research on LOAD, our thinking matured. We now hold that the best way to prevent LOAD is within a comprehensive framework that we have labelled: Biologically and Sociologically Informed Cognitive Behavioral Technologies for the Prevention of Alzheimers. We struggled with the term *Sociologically Informed* while looking for a term to characterize the influences commerce plays in determining the chances that an older citizen will develop LOAD. Commercial interests play an extraordinarily significant role in determining whether any given citizen might develop the disease. Many commentators have expressed the idea that an individuals' lifestyle is a major factor in the development of Alzheimers. However, their concept of lifestyles usually did not include the influence that drug companies and other allied companies (e.g., media) hold over people's lives.

Activities of our commercial world can yield great benefits, as well as great harm. This is no mystery, money indexes value and power. Commerce is the vehicle for the transfer of money. Governing bodies of nearly every modern nation constantly struggle to govern commercial activities of drug companies; which at times are not in the interest of the consumer.

There is a special interest in controlling drugs because (a) they are small enough to be taken regularly, (b) often easily manufactured and marketed, (c) when used improperly drugs can be and often are poisonous, (d) can be addictive, a distributor's dream, (e) a lot of money can be made selling drugs, and (f) they can be life-saving, consequently no one needing a drug to control a deadly disease should be denied access to the drug. Because all of this is bound up with extensive commercial activities, drugs are a major feature of modern life. Our premise is that an informed citizen should be aware of how drug and the natural-drug-supplement manufacturers and distributors attempt to manipulate our lives in the service of making money. Their interests in making money often overrides their interest in public health.

This book is the product of a lot of work other than that of the authors. We are grateful for the overall structure of a major research university, Rensselaer Polytechnic Institute, that provides means to do scholarly activities. We particularly thank all of the students that have taken an interest in the Project. In particular, we than Dylan Z Taylor who has assumed the role of a major colleague in the development of the work associated with the goal of preventing Alzheimer's disease. We are particularly grateful to Mohammed O. Moftah whose work in developing a salient website has been critical to the Project. We thank Ropa Denga with her editorial assistance with portions of this book.

Paula Monahan, you make my (Larry's) life easier by being helpful, thank you. And, we both thank Lawrence D. Reid for his companionship and partnership.

Contents

Preface v
Contents viii
Introduction 1
Kinds of Sleep Disorders 1
Insomnia: A Risk for the Development of Alzheimer's Disease 2
There are Two Kinds of Sleep, Both Important 5
    On the Content of Dreams 12
Sleeping and Learning 13
Sleep and the Brain's Metabolic Waste 15
"Sleeping Pills" Can Be Part of a Larger Problem. 20
    Drug-Treatments for Insomnia 20
        Prescription Hypnotics 21
        The Z-drugs 28
        An Orexin Antagonist 33
    Some Prescription Drugs are Surely Safer than Others. 38
    OTC Hypnotic Drugs and Dietary Supplements 39
Some Final Comments about the Risks of Sleeping Pills 41
Issues of Polypharmacy 48
    Prescription Drugs 51
    OTC Drugs 54
    The Dietary Supplement Market 56
    The Anticholinergic Burden 62
    Managing Polypharmacy 65
    Drug-Withdrawal 65
Commerce Associated with Sleeping 69
    Vested Interests 70
        At the Law-Making Level 70
        At the Drug-Company Level 73
        At the FDA Level 78
Integrated Cognitive Behavioral Therapy (CBT) for Alzheimers 80
Cognitive Behavioral Technologies for Insomnia (CBTs-I) 84

  Science on Biologically and Sociological Informed CBTs-I 85
  Fundamentals of CBTs-I 87
  A Noteworthy Feature of CBTs-I 89
There is Value to Regular Medical Checkups 91
CBTs-I 91
  Question 92
  Answer 92
  Consultation 92
  Participants' Questions 96
  Chronic Insomnia 97
Arrange Your Bedroom for Sleep 99
  Questions 99
  Answers 100
  Consultation 100
    Lighting 101
    Avoid Using Electronics Before Bedtime 101
    Temperature 102
    Clean Air 103
    Comfortable Bedding 103
The Skill to Relax on Cue 103
  Technique to Relax on Cue 104
Sleep and Anxiety 108
  Bed-bedroom Phobias 109
  Questions 109
  Answers 110
  Consultation 110
  Managing a Bed-Bedroom Phobia 113
    Counter-Conditioning 114
    A Daytime way to Reduce Sleep Anxiety 116
  Your Time Just Before Sleeping 117
  Fearing Loss of Consciousness 118
  Change the Stimuli Associated with Insomnia 121
Establish a Schedule for Optimal Sleep 122
  Questions 123

    Answers 124
    Consultation 125
        The Value of this Routine 127
Other Issues that Might Need Attention 128
    Waking Up in the Middle of a Sleep-Period 128
    Exercise and Unusual Exercises 129
    Anxiety and Depression 130
    Thought-stopping 131
    Mindfulness 132
Summary 133
References 135
Appendix 141
About the Authors 148

Introduction

Sleep is essential. A 72-hour period of sleep-deprivation puts us into a state that makes it almost impossible to stay awake another minute. During the last hours of a 72-hour period of sleep deprivation, a person will be less alert, less competent, and probably irritable and unhappy.

Nearly everyone sleeps sometime within a 24-hour period. Some folks find sleep pleasureable and look forward to repeating it daily. Others view sleep as a necessary nuisance. A few thinks of sleep as an obstacle depriving them of the pleasures they might enjoy if they did not need it. Regardless of how we might view sleep, sleep we must!

Even though we spend about a third of our lives preparing to sleep, sleeping, and arousing from sleep, the scientific community lacks a full understanding of the physiology of sleeping. This does not mean that we are ignorant about sleep; we know a lot about sleep. However, the process of sleeping seems to have a complexity that we have yet to fully understand (more on this later).

Kinds of Sleep Disorders

Some diagnostic manuals for disease list 10 kinds of sleep disorders. Among the 10 listed are insomnia (includes interrupted sleep), sleep apnea (associated with difficulty breathing during sleep), sleep walking, nightmares, and other rare sleep disorders.

By far the most prevalent sleep disorder is insomnia. A prominent sleep researcher defined insomnia this way: "(1) difficulty falling asleep, staying asleep or nonrestorative sleep; (2) this difficulty is present despite adequate opportunity and circumstance to sleep; (3) this impairment in sleep is associated with daytime impairment or distress; and (4) this sleep difficulty occurs at least 3 times per week and has been a problem for at least 1 month."[1(pS7)]

Various surveys from around the world tabulate the prevalence of insomnia. In North America and Europe about 30% of adults report experiencing persisting insomnia at some period during their lifetime. Insomnia appears to be more common among older citizens and more common among women than men.[1]

Insomnia: A Risk for the Development of Alzheimer's Disease

This book focuses on insomnia because it is the most common sleep disorder and a risk-factor for the development of late-onset Alzheimer's disease.

Most citizens of prosperous nations who reach the age of retirement (about the age of about 65 years old) can have the reasonable expectation of living another three decades if they can avoid the most common deadly diseases. Among those common diseases is Alzheimer's disease. To meet the expectation of living well into the 9th decade, it will be necessary to do activities preventing the most common diseases of aging. There are lifestyles conducive to healthy aging and there are lifestyles that promote fast aging and early death.

An essential feature of a healthy lifestyle is developing the habit of getting a *good night's sleep*. The real test of whether a period of sleep is healthy, or not so healthy, is how one feels upon awakening. After a good night of sleep, an individual is rested, clear-headed, and somewhat ready to begin a day of activities. After a bad night of sleep, an individual does not feel rested, seems unable to function as well as they should, gets tired easily, and has trouble thinking well.

Our perspective: Toward the beginning of one's retirement-decades is a time to act to lower the risk of developing Alzheimer's disease. Further our understanding of the disease indicates that retirees can do that; that is, they can prevent Alzheimer's disease from ruining the last decades of their lives. Retirees can do that by engaging in activities that protect against the development of Alzheimer's disease. Activities that prevent Alzheimer's disease also protect against other causes of premature death (e.g., cardio-vascular diseases).

It is painfully apparent that there is no way of restoring the lost brain tissue of advanced Alzheimer's disease. We have yet to discover a way of stopping the insidious progression of the disease which eventually leaves many retirees without a mature mind and helpless (i.e., becoming demented). The obvious conclusion: Prevention is the only available "cure" for Alzheimer's disease.

This book focuses on two essential risks that need to be corrected to prevent Alzheimer's disease: insomnia and the intake of certain drugs. The good news: Insomnia can be successfully treated. Further, Alzheimers can be successfully prevented by engaging activities that promote a healthy brain as one ages; which includes routinely getting a *good night's sleep.* To repeat the bad news: Alzheimer's disease, once clearly underway, currently cannot be halted from progressing to dementia. To repeat the good news: The risk of insomnia can be reduced thereby significantly reducing the risks of developing Alzheimer's disease.

Also, we are learning that some commonly taken drugs are risky, particularly when taken continuously. They are risky because they have problematic side-effects. Concordantly, they put individuals at risk for Alzheimer's disease.[1] Consequently, those drugs should not be taken regularly.

The writing that immediately follows this paragraph discusses in some detail the biology of sleep and the use of drugs to control sleep disorders. The discussion of the biology of sleep is a prelude to a description of an effective non-drug treatment of insomnia and related issues. The part presenting the details of managing chronic insomnia *begins* with the title "Integrated Cognitive Behavioral Therapy (CBT) for Alzheimers." That part presents a way to treat insomnia in a safe, healthy way. If you are eager to start treating insomnia, you might immediately turn to the treatment-section of the book. However, if you take the time to read and understand the first part of the book, you will gain an understanding of why we recommend the preferred treatment for insomnia and related problems.

There are Two Kinds of Sleep, Both Important

The scientific study of sleep did not really begin until the 20th century. Of course, throughout history, there were many discussions about why we sleep and the content of dreams.

An important step toward the scientific study of sleep was made by Hans Berger, a 19th century scientist. Berger was the first to get a record of gross changes in the ongoing electrical activity of the human brain revealed by recording-electrodes placed on the scalp. Those recordings became known as an electroencephalogram (EEG). Now, modern and improved ways of recording EEGs continue to be useful for studying sleep.

An EEG is a high fidelity recording of neural activity occurring in the brain by measuring small electrical changes using electrodes placed on the scalp. A recording of these moment by moment changes is made by an ink-pen that moves up and down reflecting changes in the activity of the brain, on a moving sheet of paper (see the accompany figure).

The first observations of this stream of electrical changes were novel and there were discussions about what they might signify. The only logical conclusion was that they represented a feature of the brain at work.

Among the first well-established conclusions was that one pattern of activity characterized being awake while another pattern characterized being asleep. When an individual was in a coma, the EEG appeared rather flat. When an individual was dead, there were no changes in an EEG (hence the phrase "flat lined" signifying death).

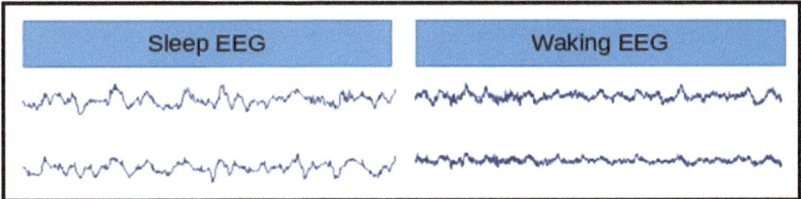

A depiction of two kinds of EEGs, one typical of sleep and one typical of being awake. The sleep pattern is of larger waves with lower frequency (called alpha waves) and the awake, alert pattern is indexed by high frequency fast waves (called beta waves).

A physiologist, Nathaniel Klietman (1895-1999) of the University of Chicago, spent his career studying sleep. At the time, few others shared his interest in sleep. Klietman is considered the father of sleep-research. He famously explored whether our circadian rhythms were a function of the presence of daylight during the day and how sleep is affected by the absence of daylight during nighttime. To study that, he and a colleague spent many days inside a completely dark cave using only artificial lighting. They learned that the marked tendency to be sleepy during the night was sustained even though it was not apparent in the cave what time of the 24-hour day it was. The circadian pattern of sleep was robust.

Klietman and a colleague, Eugene Aserinsky, set to work studying sleep throughout the night with an EEG machine more sophisticated than that of Berger. Aserinsky used his son Armond as his subject. Armond spent his sleep-time in the lab while his father recorded his EEG throughout the night. The father noticed that while his son looked like he was sound asleep, his EEG indicated he was awake. He went to his son and asked him, "why are you awake?", and his son awoke and replied, "I was dreaming." He then observed multiple EEG readings indicating wakefulness occurring during sleep. It became apparent, over the course of an ordinary period of sleep, there were periods of awake-like EEGs during which dreaming or mental activity occurred. The waves recorded during these periods came to be known as beta waves.

When recording-electrodes are placed near the corners of the eyes, electrical signals generated by the muscles that move the eyes can be observed and recorded. Eugene noticed that eye movements and brain waves indicative of being awake (beta waves), tended to occur together. The movement of the eyes under closed lids can be observed without the use of a machine; however, the recordings made it possible to record the movement in a dark room and notice their exact time and duration. It became apparent that beta waves, rapid eye movements and dreaming typically occur at the same time during sleep.

Given the relationship among beta waves (awake-like EEGs), rapid eye movement and dreaming, the name of this circumstance became known as rapid eye movement sleep, i.e., *REM sleep*.   Other patterns of EEG recordings are called *nonREM sleep.* This label of REM sleep and nonREM sleep (rather than dream sleep and non-dream sleep) was chosen because similar findings were observed in other animals like dogs and cats. One can record an animal's eye movements, but one cannot discuss their dreams with them.

These initial observations instigated a flurry of research with some important findings:

Surprisingly, we have REM-sleep periods every night at a rate of about 4 or occasionally, 5 or 6 of them. Yet, we have little awareness of this upon awakening. Of course, sometimes we experience a dream, but the experience of many nightly dreams escapes us.

Research in humans and lab-animals demonstrates that deprivation of REM-sleep can cause multiple symptoms of poor health. We, of course, know that sleep itself is necessary for good health and we now know that REM-sleep (dreaming) is also necessary.

Babies have REM sleep.

All mammals tested, and other kinds of animals, also show patterns of periods resembling REM- and nonREM-sleep.

When REM-sleep is repeatedly reduced, there is an apparent drive to obtain REM-sleep.

This is manifest by having a REM episode early in an ensuing period of sleep.

When awakened with a reduced amount of REM-sleep, one feels tired and there are urges to sleep.

The figure depicts the typical circadian rhythm of an adult human being. The individual begins sleep just after just after 22 hours and sleeps about 8 hours. Within the population, there is considerable variation of the length of time of sleeping. Variations in gray indicate Non-REM sleep. Red signifies periods of REM sleep. The graph was created by Dylan Z Taylor.

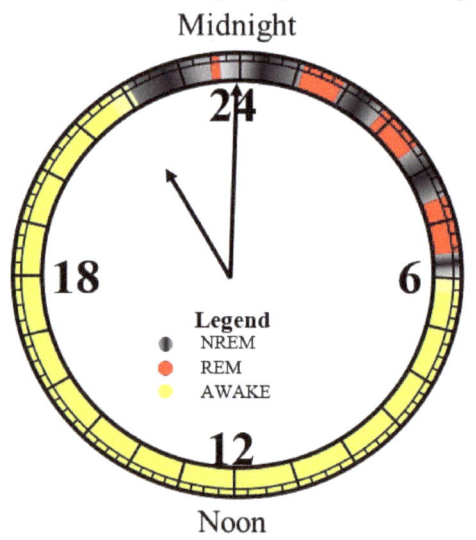

Important implications followed from knowing the new facts about sleep. For example, any circumstance that might interfere with REM-sleep is apt to be disturbing. We will return to this line of thinking as we discuss treatments for sleep-problems.

A similar implication: Disturbances of a pattern of healthy sleep (e.g., not having adequate amounts of both REM- and nonREM-sleep) might be a causal event in other disorders. Since we are not particularly aware of a lack of REM-sleep, it is not obvious that a problem may be due to a lack of REM-sleep. Any tiredness, for example, is likely to be attributed to something else. Also, medical professionals often do not ask about sleep; therefore, problems of sleep are not considered when making recommendations for treatments. Of course, sometimes an individual may offer the diagnosis that they are sleepy and tired during the day and report that they do not regularly have a good night's sleep.

A reduced amount of sleep or reduced REM-sleep causes one to wake up feeling tired and groggy. The immediate solution, often, is to take a stimulant such as a large dose of caffeine. Or, even taking a dose of a drug such as Adderall (amphetamine) or similar stimulants (a really poor choice is cocaine). This is a temporary fix. If done repeatedly, serious problems will emerge eventually.

Drinking multiple alcoholic beverages exacerbates the tiredness one feels from poor sleep. An initial drink is often stimulating, but more than one usually induces fatigue and some signs of being drunk. Lethargy (due to poor sleep, such as reduced REM sleep) and drunkenness can combine with sleep deprivation to reduce alertness such that it is not safe to drive a car. Drinking after work is a staple of modern life for many individuals.

Sleep deprivation and the intake of alcoholic beverages together produce impaired judgement and a reduction in well-coordinated behavior. In other words, being sleepy and intoxicated can lead to accidents; even fatal accidents. For retirees, being sleepy and intoxicated increases the risk of falls and, hence, broken bones.

The take-away message from the understanding of the importance of sleep is that we should do nothing that might interfere with our dreaming, our REM sleep. After a few comments about the content of dreams, we turn our attention to understanding the functions of sleep.

On the Content of Dreams

There has always been controversy about the meaning of the contents of dreaming. Throughout history dreams were thought to be messages from supernatural beings or forecasts of the future or recalled past episodes of life that were lost to memory, etc. However, there has been considerable effort to discern the meanings of dreams by those treating patients with psychological disorders. The consensus is little was gained from that activity. It could be that dreams are indeed meaningless with respect to specific content, but meaningful with respect to sustaining a healthy physiology of the brain.

One idea is that dreams are a way of shifting fluids throughout the brain so that the brain gets washed throughout nearly every night and the dream is merely a byproduct of that physiology.[2]

Despite a lack of apparent progress concerning the content of dreams, there's still ongoing research on dreams. For example, one relatively new idea is that the complexity of dreaming tends to mute the memory of aversive events.[3]

Sleeping and Learning

Experimental psychologists are learning about learning, hence about habit-formation. Within that framework, it has been discovered that the consolidation of newly learned material is a process associated with sleep. In other words, lessons learned while awake are further processed during sleep.

During sleep, our experiences are consolidated such that we have memory of the *important events* of the day, i.e., events that signal pleasure or pain.

The experience of pleasure or pain (and the multiple varieties of each) is basically a process that evolved to sustain life sufficiently to propagate the species. In other words, evolution equipped us with a system to guide our behavior so that it is adaptive. We seek pleasure. Pleasurable events typically sustain us (e.g., eating when hungry, drinking when thirsty, sleeping when sleepy, not being bored, etc.). We avoid that which is painful and scary, hence protecting us from harm. Now, we all know that this rather crude way of directing our behavior is not sufficient to sustain living for a long time. We are also equipped with the ability to think wisely.

It is truly sobering to come to the realization that our development of being able to think wisely is so dependent upon regularly sleeping well. Processes occurring during sleep allow habits to be formed. It follows from common knowledge, as well as the scientific study of long-term memory and habit-formation, that any event that might disturb sleep might also disturb memory of events of the day before and hence disturb the refinement of behaviors called habits or skills.

In brief, sleep is different than resting, it is a vital part of maturing and the refinement of our ability to efficiently adapt to life's reoccurring circumstances.

What we know about learning and sleep does not seem to be the full explanation for why we sleep. Yes, sleep facilitates the formation of long-term memories; however, there are other physiologies that appear to be happening during sleep.

Sleep and the Brain's Metabolic Waste

One of the most important functions of sleep is to cleanse the brain of debris. Here we will take a somewhat more detailed look at how this occurs.

A well-functioning brain needs an enormous amount of glucose and oxygen to provide the energy necessary to keep neurons in a ready-state, i.e., ready to transfer information. Energy is also needed to transfer and process information throughout the brain and coordinate the functions of the body. This need is met by a constant and plentiful supply of blood. That is: The blood leaving the heart and reaching the brain is a relatively large part of the heart's output. An adult human brain weighs about 3 pounds and the rest of the body, on average, about 150 pounds; however, the brain receives up to 15% of the blood leaving the heart.

Since the brain has little to no capacity to store energy, it needs a constant supply of blood. Any disruption of the blood-supply to the brain lasting more than a few minutes can cause serious brain damage. It follows: To have a healthy brain while aging, it is necessary to have a healthy cardio-vascular system.

Having a healthy cardio-vascular system involves eating a healthy diet and having a habit of regular physical exercise. Diet and exercise are topics for a different place and a different time.

Here, we address a consequence of the brain's high rate of energy use; that is, the brain generates waste. It is, therefore, necessary to regularly cleanse the brain of that metabolic waste.

The brain and the rest of the body have different ways of eliminating the waste that usually accumulates in the fluid between cells (interstitial fluid). It turns out that some substances floating along in blood vessels can and must exit the vessels along with blood plasma.

In every part of the body (except the brain), there are lymph vessels close to nearly every cell of the body. Fluid exiting the blood vessels is collected in lymph vessels of the lymphatic circulatory system. The lymphatic circulatory system has the essential functions of aiding in the elimination of wastes and recirculating fluid pushed out of blood vessels, thereby sustaining the homeostasis of maintaining fluid-balances throughout the body.

The fluid draining into lymph vessels contains metabolic waste as well as other substances which are to be processed and eliminated or re-circulated and used in other parts of the body. As this happens, the fluid between cells of the body are eventually cleansed of waste. You can think of the waste-products as garbage and the lymph system as the garbage collector that sends the garbage to be processed and eventually eliminated.

Some of the products that might leak from peripheral blood vessels are lethal to the cells of the brain. Consequently, there is a blood-brain-barrier that protects the brain from some of the stuff circulating throughout the vascular system. The arteries of the brain only allow substances needed to nourish the brain to leave the arteries and go into neurons and other cells of the brain.

Unlike the rest of the body, there are no lymph vessels scattered throughout the brain. The brain has a unique way of managing accumulation of waste in the fluids between cells and in sustaining the fluid-balances that are absolutely necessary for a brain surrounded by a hard, inflexible skull. There must be a balance between the heart pumping large amounts of fluid into the skull, hence brain, to be matched (balanced) by an equal amount of fluid leaving the brain in order to sustain the integrity of the tissue of the brain.

Most of the issues associated with maintaining a balance of fluids entering and leaving the brain are handled by the amount of arterial blood entering the brain and the veins carrying fluids out of the brain. However, that artery to vein fluid-exchange does not account for how waste, such proteins, are carried out of the fluid (interstitial fluid) between neurons.

One of the cardinal events in the development of Alzheimer's disease is an accumulation of proteins in the interstitial fluid surrounding the cells of the brain. Among the proteins that tend to accumulate in the brain's interstitial fluid is a protein made nearly continuously called amyloid beta.

The brain produces its own interstitial fluid called cerebral spinal fluid; which is filtered blood plasma. The blood-brain-barrier prevents toxic materials that might be in blood from making their way to the brain. The brain handles cellular waste and other products produced by neurons by delivering such to the interstitial fluid where it then flows out of the brain and into the lymph vessels surrounding the brain.

Neurons of the brain produce a protein called amyloid beta (also known beta amyloid) which has important functions. However, if beta amyloid accumulates in the interstitial fluid of the brain it can form clumps called amyloid plaques. When these clumps become large and numerous, they can be toxic to neurons. Just how they become toxic has not been detailed;

however, it is known that it is not a good thing for the amyloid plaques to grow and accumulate in the fluid of the brain. In fact, the best supported theory of the development of Alzheimers holds that an accumulation of amyloid plaques is a cause of Alzheimers.[5]

Here is the point that we wish to make: *The removal of garbage from the brain is best done during healthy sleep.*[4] It appears that during the day when the brain is working to adjust behavior to the circumstances we are experiencing, the garbage tends to accumulate and is not adequately washed away from the cells of the brain by the movement of the brain's fluid as it moves out of the brain. However, during sleep there are changes in the brain allowing for more efficient garbage-removal which prevents an accumulation of amyloid beta and other proteins. It follows from this biology that *poor sleep is a risk-factor for the development of Alzheimers*.

Also, it is important to know that there are both dangerous and safe ways of "correcting" poor sleep. Obviously, it is prudent to choose safe methods. The safest way to correct poor sleep is also the way to sustain healthy sleep on a daily basis. The rest of this book is a caution against dangerous ways of correcting poor sleep and a discussion on safe ways of getting a good night's sleep.

"Sleeping Pills" Can Be Part of a Larger Problem.

Drugs marketed to treat insomnia are called *Hypnotics.* To put the problems related to hypnotics in context, we will present some of the broader issues associated with the development and marketing of drugs in the USA.

Drug-Treatments for Insomnia

There is a rational distinction between brief instances of insomnia and chronic insomnia (sustained, reoccurring insomnia). Brief instances usually are corrected by merely providing a good opportunity to sleep during the next day, or over the next couple of days. The problems associated with chronic insomnia are clearly serious and often are associated with a host of co-morbid disorders. Further, chronic insomnia is often difficult to treat sufficiently well to restore ordinary, healthy sleep. Given the difficulty in correcting chronic insomnia, drugs have been developed to treat chronic insomnia. First, we will address issues associated with prescription hypnotics. Subsequently, we will address the OTC (Over the Counter) drugs and dietary supplements used to treat insomnia.

About 9 million USA citizens, during any recent year, take a prescription drug for insomnia, and many more take OTC drugs and dietary supplements.[5] Citizens over 65 years old take more of these drugs than younger citizens. Pharmaceutical companies stoke this large, steady, profitable market with sophisticated, highly tested and developed advertising, featuring quick fixes for what can be enduring problems.

Prescription Hypnotics

We will discuss, at some length, the prescription hypnotics that have been marketed and used for the last half century or so and a novel hypnotic (Belsomra) introduced recently.

Most prescription hypnotics are members of the following classes: barbiturates, benzodiazepines, and benzodiazepine-like drugs (Z drugs). There are different drugs within each class. The different drugs within a class often differ from one another by being either short-acting or long-acting. The Z-drugs were deliberately developed to be short acting, that is act only during the beginning of the sleep cycle. There are over 20 benzodiazepines (or drugs acting similarly to benzodiazepines) approved by the FDA (Food and Drug Administration) to be prescribed in the USA and are available for marketing. Many of these drugs have multiple brand names.

There are a wide variety of hypnotics in the OTC and dietary supplement market, surely more brands than active ingredients.

When taken, all variants within each class and all the classes of hypnotics visibly produce some level of sedation. Whether these drugs are used as a hypnotic or an anti-anxiety drug, they have similar actions in the brain and present some of the same problems.

These drugs differ in how the body handles them in various ways. One way is how fast they are metabolized (broken down) which, in turn, determines how long they circulate throughout the body, including the brain. As long as the drugs circulate throughout the brain, they can repeatedly influence the actions of brain cells. Most hypnotics, however, have similar actions on neurons of the brain which is the topic of the next few paragraphs.

Virtually all neurons of the brain have receptors for both excitatory and inhibitory neurotransmitters. The interaction between excitation and inhibition regulates the eventual transfer of information from one neuron to the next. An analogy that is not totally apt, but one we are familiar with: the excitatory neuro-transmitter acting on a receptor for that neurotransmitter is analogous to making a car go forward by pushing on the gas pedal. Further, the more pressure on the pedal (giving the engine more gas) the more likely the car will move forward. The inhibitory neuro-transmitter is analogous to putting on the brakes or the inertia of going uphill. The interplay between excitation and inhibition determines whether a car moves forward.

To extend the analogy a bit, a neuron is like a car that has just been started, i.e., it is ready to move. The engine is running and using fuel and there is exhaust (waste) being generated (recall the section of the book on "Sleep and the Brain's Metabolic Waste). A car with a running engine but not getting sufficient gas to move forward is analogous to a neuron's state of being ready for action (step on the gas and go forward).

The major excitatory neuro-transmitter is glutamate, an amino acid. The major inhibitory neuro-transmitter is GABA (short for **g**amma **a**mino**b**utyric **a**cid). Practically all neurons have receptors for these two major neurotransmitters. Nearly all the prescription hypnotics (and anti-anxiety drugs) act on the receptors for GABA (specifically the $GABA_A$ receptor). They do not act like GABA, but rather facilitate the actions of GABA. Hence, they produce sedation by inhibiting many neurons of the brain.

Interestingly, barbiturates, benzodiazepines and Z-drugs act on slightly different parts of the GABA receptor to produce the facilitation of GABA, hence sedation. This feature accounts for the fact that these drugs' effects can combine, when taken concurrently, to produce more sedation than either might alone. As we learned more about the mechanism accounting for the benzodiazepines (i.e., the Valium-like drugs) and the barbiturates' actions, we learned that the ethanol in alcoholic beverages also acts much the same way as these two kinds of drugs and does so by acting at the GABA receptor (or put differently, the benzodiazepines act similarly to drinking alcoholic beverages).

There are over a hundred other neuro-transmitters. Many of them might be better called neuro-modulators. Neuro-modulators work like the thermostats in your home, i.e., they set the level at which a furnace turns on and off. Regarding neurons, a neuro-modulator sets how much overall excitation (the interaction of both excitatory and inhibitory neuro-transmitters) is necessary for a neuron to transfer information.

As if you did not know already, the brain is a very complex system. Drugs that facilitate widespread inhibition across nearly the entire brain are not apt to be specific for any given problem.

An unfortunate feature of barbiturates is that their fatally toxic doses and their desired doses (therapeutic doses) are very close to one another. Given the potential lethality of barbiturates, the choice of a drug to control insomnia and anxiety became a benzodiazepine or benzodiazepine-like drug. These drugs' toxic doses are large; hence, they are safer in terms of their immediate toxic effects. We guess that no prescriptions are currently written for a barbiturate to be given to treat insomnia (they are prescribed for other disorders and uses). Given this circumstance, we will only discuss the hypnotics used currently, i.e., the benzdiazepines, benzodiazepine-like drugs or Z-drugs and Belsomra.

Recall, our discussion of REM-sleep and that REM-sleep is essential for good health. It turns out, that benzodiazepines, barbiturates and alcohol each and all reduce REM-sleep to nearly nil provided these drugs are circulating throughout the brain. The basis for this is that all of them enhance GABA's inhibitory actions. Given this problematic feature, the idea arose to develop short acting hypnotics that would help induce sleep but not last long enough to reduce all REM-sleep. An example of this concept is the development of the Z-drugs (more on this later).

The net effect of a benzodiazepine is to facilitate the unconsciousness that starts a period of sleep, but that has the additional effect of suppressing the REM sleep usually occurring toward the end of a sleep-period. A suppression of REM sleep has the effect of leaving an individual groggy and less alert upon awakening. This state, then, might be medicated with a lot of coffee (caffeine) which might temporarily take care of the grogginess.

However, a lot of coffee will not prevent feeling tired in the afternoon. To correct that afternoon let-down, some individuals seek stronger stimulants than coffee (e.g., an amphetamine or a worse choice, cocaine) which might then leave them unable to quickly go to sleep which then leads them to take a benzodiazepine to facilitate going to sleep. As you can discern, this is a condition for a vicious cycle of medication which has a host of other side-effects and surely many of which are unhealthy (e.g., a stressed cardio-vascular system). Unfortunately, we do not have sufficient research to indicate if there is some recovery of ability to have REM sleep after this cycle of medication. It is unlikely, however, that all REM sleep is abolished by sustained intake of hypnotics. Nevertheless, the cycle of medications (drugs to get to sleep and then drugs to stay awake during the time one should be awake) is surely antithetical to being healthy.

There is a disturbing study providing evidence for the following conclusion: The regular use of the commonly prescribed hypnotics and anti-anxiety drugs, the benzodiazepines, increases the risk of developing Alzheimers.[6] The researches used the data of drug-prescriptions in Canada where all prescriptions are tabulated (a feature of socialized medicine, i.e., the government pays for medicines that are prescribed and that provides a record of virtually all drug-prescriptions). They then formed two groups of elderly citizens: *one group* during a 6-year period had been prescribed one or more of the benzodiazepines as probably a sleep-aid or as an anti-anxiety drug. The *other group* were similar in age and in 20 other characteristics but were not prescribed benzodiazepines. They then tracked the health records for these two large groups (over 1700 patients in each) for five years while tabulating instances of Alzheimers and particularly Alzheimers dementia. The results indicate that the risk of developing Alzheimers was about 47% greater among those prescribed benzodiazepines compared to those who were not.

Note the study showing that benzodiazepine-use was associated with the development of Alzheimers merely shows a correlation and does not prove causality. Nevertheless, the correlation is large and statistically meaningful (too large to occur by chance). When they looked at other possible causes, such as having depression, they found that such did not change the risk. The habitual use of benzodiazepines, particularly at high doses, can evidently condition the brain so that Alzheimers is more likely to develop earlier than it would otherwise. Also, the risk was greater when the used-benzodiazepine was one of the long-acting ones (examples being Valium and Librium). The authors of the study pointed out that other similar studies with a smaller number of patients found a similar association.

Prescription hypnotics, at their recommended doses, cause a person to fall into unconscious faster than they would normally and stay unconscious for a period. They do not induce sleep. True sleep is a rather complex process. One complexity is that there are cycles of non-REM and REM sleep which occur in a systematic order in natural sleep that does not occur with the state produced by prescription hypnotic drugs. Note again, benzodiazepines and benzodiazepine-like drugs reduce REM sleep, interfere with memory consolidation, and can be part of polypharmacy.

The Z-drugs

The long-acting benzodiazepines, the active ingredient in many sleeping pills, block REM sleep which, as we have learned, is not a healthy outcome. To develop a pill that does not completely block REM sleep, short-acting benzodiazepines-like compounds were developed. They are zolpidem (Ambien), zaleplon (Sonata), zopiclone (Imovane) and eszopiclone (Lunesta). They are referred to as Z-drugs (rather than benzodiazepine-like drugs) because they all have Zs in their name.[7] They are all short acting and accentuate the actions of the neurotransmitter GABA and produce widespread neuro-inhibition.

When the Z-drugs were first introduced they were widely adopted, in part, because they were skillfully marketed to be superior to the longer acting benzodiazepines. However, it appears that the Z-drugs have as many problems as the longer acting benzodiazepines.

It should be noted that the consensus recommendation of nearly all sleep experts is that prescription hypnotics acting at GABA receptors should be prescribed only for short durations, say a few days and surely not for multiple months. Despite this consensus view, the reality is the contrary. Individuals often take them regularly and they are prescribed regularly. When taken regularly, there is an issue of how to quit using them. It is a problem because, there are likely to be withdrawal symptoms such as anxiety, return of insomnia, irritability, and tremor and muscle spasms that are manifest as insomnia when dosing is stopped.

A recent review (appearing in 2017), by Brandt and Leong,[7] explored the data on the relationship of benzodiazepines and Z-drugs to a variety of disease and disorders. The list of potential disorders that these hypnotics might cause or exacerbate is extensive ranging from simple falls to deadly diseases such as cancer.

They concluded that there is sufficient evidence from epidemiological and experimental research to conclude there is a strong, causal connection between hypnotic drug-use and motor vehicle crashes, and falls (particularly, hip fractures). These drugs induce psychomotor impairment which is clearly dose-related. Also, drug overdoses leading to death are often related, without question, to the intake of these hypnotics in combination with other sedating drugs or with intake of alcoholic beverages.

A recent article found that when retirees take benzodiazepines or Z-drugs, they are more likely to suffer from hip fractures.[8] Among those suffering from a broken hips, about a quarter of them die within a year of the accident. Others suffer considerable loss of health and incapacity. The findings also indicate that benzodiazepines or Z-drugs are equally risky when it comes to hip fractures. Individuals are at the highest risk when they first start taking the drug. Now, this should not be a surprise, given what we know about these drugs. They induce effects resembling alcoholic beverages, due to similar actions at the GABA receptor. When first given to an unsuspecting retiree, they produce drunkenness which is a disturbance of psychomotor ability (everyone knows drinkers, even experienced drinkers, often stager when walking and have more accidents). Given some time, drinkers who drink regularly learn to walk better when drunk so that they reduce their chances of accidents, but that learning often does not overcome the total effects of being intoxicated.

According to Brandt and Leong,[7] the evidence clearly supports the conclusion that these hypnotics increase the chances of a fall sufficiently severe to cause hip fractures. *Taking hypnotics is dangerous because it increases the risk of serious accidents.*

Brandt and Leong reviewed the association of hypnotics to increases (a) in infections probably due to interference with the immune system, (b) pancreatitis, disease of the pancreas, (c) respiratory disease exacerbation, (d) dementia, including Alzheimers, and (e) cancer, and took a very conservative stance. They indicated that the research was not yet definitive despite, in some cases, controlled animal studies indicating a direct relationship between hypnotics and disease-progression.

The potential benefit of these drugs in relationship to their treatment of insomnia and anxiety disorders is not strong; in fact, these drugs are minimally effective. Further, adverse effects multiply if these drugs are taken chronically. There are safer alternatives that are equally effective and often shown to be superior to dosing with hypnotics (the alternative is discussed at length subsequently).

Brandt and Leong's conclusions: widely sold hypnotics surely increase the risks of (a) accidents (falls, and auto crashes), especially among retirees and (b) deaths by overdosing.

They also discussed the question of whether the use of hypnotics might (likely or maybe) increase the risks of leading causes of death (cancer, respiratory diseases, and dementia) as indicated in some research. Their conclusion is that there is only weak to modestly strong evidence to support that hypnotic-use might be involved with these serious diseases. In the face of this, Brandt and Leong's advice is to do more research in case we find that, in fact, hypnotics do not increase infections, but infections are more closely related to some other factor "merely" exacerbated by hypnotics.

One might applaud Brandt and Leong for being cautious about concluding that these drugs may increase the risk of major diseases. Nevertheless, their cautiousness seems to sanction the continuance of clearly dangerous practices until there is finally no shadow of a doubt about the dangerousness of the unacceptable practice of widely prescribing hypnotics. Recall, they concluded, without reservation, that the use of hypnotics increased the risks of auto-accidents and falls.

The vested interests of the local drug store, the media who profit from sustained advertising, and the large drug companies are generally happy with the institutional, ingrained habits of either ignoring the seriousness of poor sleep and ignoring the widespread use of hypnotic drugs despite their marginal benefit and clearly harmful effects. Their general "solution" to similar problems (say the issue of smoking cigarettes and lung cancer) is to claim there is not yet sufficient science to support widespread disturbances in the way things are being done. The common "solution" is to do more research when in fact more research, although valuable, is not a remedy for addressing currently dangerous institutional habits that foster individual habits that are likely to be disease-producing causing premature death.

Fortunately, most (actually nearly all) individuals can by their own actions effectively deal with their own problems of insomnia without the help of hypnotics. They can do that because their own physiology will help them accomplish the goal of healthy sleep. All that is necessary is a little help specifying how to do that (much of which is common sense) and the understanding that it can be done with some effort.

An Orexin Antagonist

A novel sleep-aid was developed and marketed after the discovery of an area of the brain that produces two neuro-modulators involved with regulating the day-night rhythm. Consequently, these neuro-modulators affect both sleep and appetite. The discovery of this small, but highly influential, area of the brain was made possible by the modern technological advances of molecular biology. The discovery was made by two laboratories: One from the University of Texas, Southwestern Medical Center and made by a team of 21 scientists, including Masashi Yanagisawa.[9] The other by a team of 15 scientists, whose lead authors Luia de Lecea and Thomas Kilduff were associated with The Scripps Research Institute and Stanford University.[10]

The gist of the two original articles and the research that followed: There are about 10,000 to 20,000 neurons in a small area of the hypothalamus (this is truly a small number with respect to the very large number of neurons, about 100 billion, in the brain). These neurons secret two neuro-modulators (both peptides) into synapses throughout the brain. These two peptides interact with receptors on a wide array of neurons in many different areas of the brain.

One function of these orexin neurons seems to be associated with arousal from sleep and sustained wakefulness. This is made manifest by the discovery that when these neurons are destroyed, (either by design in experiments with lab animals, or by genetic developments in certain dogs or humans), a disease ensues. The disease is called narcolepsy. Narcolepsy is characterized by awake-time sleepiness and lethargy and suddenly falling into a deep sleep at times outside of the bed while doing regular activities. Narcolepsy is obviously a serious disruption of an ordinary lifestyle.

In keeping with the rationale of medicinal chemists, the scientists of Merck, a large drug company, guessed that if they could develop a small molecule that could be used to make a pill to block orexin's awakening effects, hence they might have a sleep-pill to sustain a sleep-period. Again, using modern techniques, the scientists at Merck quickly developed a compound that could be an active ingredient in a sleeping pill. Then, sufficient research was done to indicate that their drug did induce sleep-like behavior, was reasonably safe to be used by humans and got it approved by the FDA for the treatment of insomnia. The FDA approved it for only temporary use and when taken at relatively small doses and as directed. The FDA did not approve larger doses because of excessive side-effects. Merck named the active ingredient, survorexant and branded the pill containing survorexant BELSOMRA.

Since it's a new kind of drug for treating insomnia and the only one of its kind, it is an expensive drug compared to what is otherwise available. The average cost is about $350.00 per prescription. Costs vary across various pharmacies, therefore the value $350.00 may be very different depending on where you might get a prescription filled.

Belsomra has some serious side-effects, including sleepiness during the day, not thinking clearly, acting strangely, being confused, upset, and while being seemingly asleep yet eating, talking, having sex or driving a car (yes, that can happen). These are all listed as serious side-effects in ads for Belsomra. They also list, in another place in the package insert, outgoing behavior, aggressive behavior, confusion, agitation, hallucinations, worsening of depression and suicidal thoughts, memory loss, anxiety, temporary inability to move or talk (sleep paralysis), and temporary weakness in your legs. They could have merely said "Belsomra can produce, but we hope not, psycho-pathology." As with other prescription medicines for insomnia, when Belsomra is taken with alcoholic beverages, the likelihood of aversive side-effects become greater.

The ad also indicates "**Do not** drive, operate heavy machinery, do anything dangerous, or do other activities that require clear thinking after taking BELSOMRA."[11] We imagine that most of the activities we engage in our modern, complex world "require clear thinking."

Note: the half-life of survorexant is roughly 12 hours which means if your take the largest dose provided commercially, 20 mg/pill, just before bed time, you will have the functional equivalent to a recommended dose of 10 mg/pill upon arousing after 8 hours in bed. That is, you "awaken" with a dose recommended to put you to sleep.

The *Clinical Practice Guideline for the Pharmacologic Treatment of Chronic Insomnia in Adults: An American Academy of Sleep Medicine Clinical Practice Guideline* suggests that clinicians use survorexant as a treatment for sleep maintenance insomnia (versus no treatment) in adults.[12] They modify the suggestion by indicating that the evidence for such a recommendation is "weak." Probably rated weak because the research was all done by the company that marketed the drug, Merck.

Consumer Reports, the independent organization that rates commercial products was funded to assess Belsomra by the "state Attorney General Consumer and Prescriber Education Grant Program which, in turn, was funded by a multistate settlement of consumer fraud claims regarding the marketing of the prescription drug Neurortin (gabapentin)."[13] (editor's note)

Consumer Reports sums their recommendation on Belsomra by saying, "It's expensive, barely helps, and poses safety concerns."[13] The safety concerns are the multiple, serious side-effects, one of which was not mentioned, that is:

a propensity for heightened appetite (something most Americans have no trouble with).

Some Prescription Drugs are Surely Safer than Others.

A recent (2018) extensive review[14] focused on drug-treatments for insomnia. As you have learned, most hypnotics do not produce restful, restorative, healthy sleep. Therefore, most available hypnotics induce next-day tiredness, reduced coordination and reduced alertness. That increases the chances of falls and motor vehicle accidents.

The authors of the 2018-review and our study of the literature lead to suggesting one hypnotic drug to use and then only rarely. There are circumstances when it is rational to help a person to get to sleep with a drug. One reason might be when insomnia might interfere with the treatment of a co-morbid disorder.

A reasonably safe drug is a short acting benzodiazepine (half-life of 1 to 2 hours) which appears to produce little if any next day sleepiness and only a few problematic side-effects with large doses. It is a prescription drug; therefore, a citizen would have to get professional advice before being able to obtain it and that is the rational circumstance. The drug is triazolam (brand name: Halcion).

Like all drugs, triazolam can induce adverse effects. A common effect is forgetfulness concerning events of the day before. One should avoid the use of the drug with intake of grapefruit juice (orange juice is O.K.) and alcoholic beverages (or other sedatives). The grapefruit juice induces effects similar to taking more of the drug than recommended and the manufacture advises against using the drug with grapefruit-products. Older citizens should take half the dose recommended for younger adults. The drug should be used temporarily and not nightly for weeks or months. Chronic use will set the conditions for withdrawal effects, the major symptom of which will probably be insomnia.[14]

OTC Hypnotic Drugs and Dietary Supplements

As a quick assessment of the size of the OTC and dietary supplement markets, we searched on Amazon, the online retailer, for how many of these kinds of products the company currently offers. The result was 96 different OTC sleep aids and 635 dietary supplements (brands) (assessment done in July 2018). Over 52% of US adults took dietary supplements from 1999-2012.[15]

There is little cost to entering the dietary supplement sleep-aid-market. Recall these products do not need to be assessed by the FDA before they are marketed, due to a change in the laws governing these products passed in 1994 (see the *vested interest* subsection on how the law was changed).

Scanning the list of ingredients of these products (surely not a complete study of this vast market), it was noted that many of them have melatonin as an active ingredient. Melatonin is a hormone produced in the pineal gland. The pineal gland is a pea-sized gland in the center of the brain thought to be the location of the soul by the French philosopher Descartes. In humans, melatonin appears to be secreted in the early hours of darkness and is thought to be associated with sleep onset and sleep maintenance. Another function of melatonin may be as an antidote to oxidative stress thereby be a neuroprotective factor.[16]

Melatonin is also produced in other places than the pineal gland (such as gut and bone marrow). Melatonin receptors are scattered throughout the body. Melatonin is also found in foods including nuts, fruits, vegetables and cereals.[16] Tryptophan, the amino acid, is the starting material for the synthesis of melatonin and circulates in blood. Given these circumstances, it seems reasonable that eating nuts, e.g., peanuts, close to bed time will probably do about as much as taking the available sleeping pills.

Sleep aids in the OTC market can have diphenhydramine, an antihistamine with considerable anticholinergic burden as a major ingredient (again, anticholinergic burden is discussed below). Although diphenhydramine will induce drowsiness and will help induce the unconsciousness at the start of sleep, its side-effect profile is too aversive to be recommended as a medicine for insomnia. Among the effects of antihistamines are that they interfere with the innate immune system of the airway and, therefore, reduce the protection of the lungs from being assaulted by bacteria and viruses that might circulate in breathed air.

Research suggests avoiding sleeping pills with the active ingredient of diphenhydramine.[16] There is considerable controversy about the use of melatonin among children and even among adults.[16]

Some Final Comments about the Risks of Sleeping Pills

Modern technology provides a powerful set of tools to learn about the effects of taking drugs. Electronic record-keeping of healthcare information, computer aided ability to extract data for analysis and modern statistical methods can be used to learn more than ever before about our prescription drugs.

Research conducted by Dr. Daniel Kripke, and his colleagues made use of such resources and published a report titled "Hypnotics' association with mortality or cancer: a matched cohort study" in 2012.[17] His findings indicate that the intake of hypnotics is associated with increased chance of dying compared to those who were not prescribed hypnotics. The more pills taken, the greater the chance of a premature death. For example, those who took more than 132 pills, per year, had over a 5 times greater chance of an early death compared to those who did not

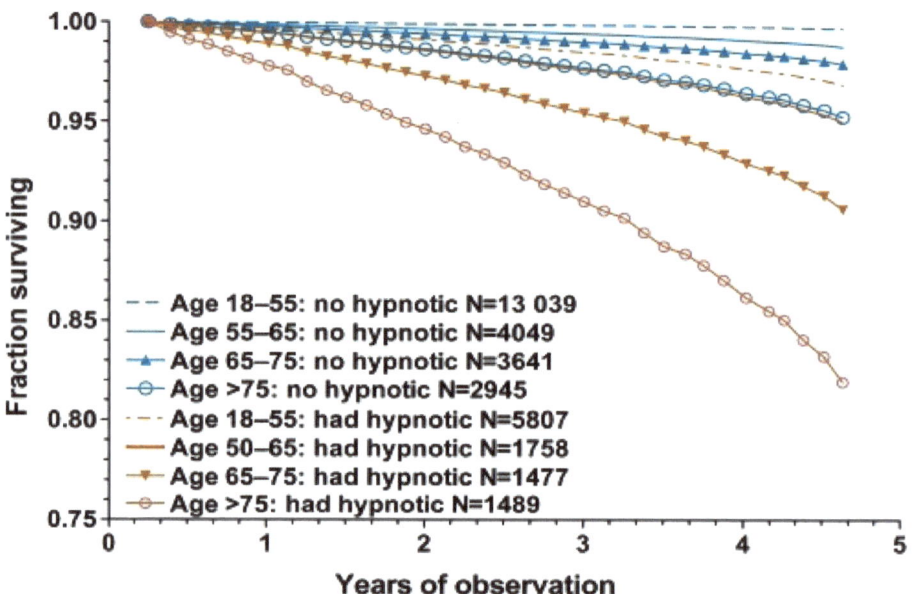

take the pills. Z-sleeping pills, temazepam and other benzodiazepines presented similar risks. Intake of a larger number of sleeping pills increased the risk of cancer. Even the intake of fewer than 18 pills per year of the Z-sleeping pills increased the risk of cancer and premature death threefold.

His study involved the electronic screening of about 224,000 patients' electronic records which included their drug-prescriptions and their diagnoses of disease. They then took all those prescribed a sleeping pill and carefully matched each of them with at least 2 persons who were not prescribed sleeping pills. Each person prescribed a pill was matched with respect to age, sex, ethnicity, marital status, body weight (BMI) and self-reported alcohol use and whether they smoked tobacco products. After all matches were arranged, they had the health records of 10,531 sleeping-pill-users and 23,676 patients who were not prescribed sleeping pills.

They then learned when each person died. As mentioned above and depicted in the accompanying graph, those prescribed sleeping pills died earlier than their matched controls. The graph depicts the data collected from Kripke's 2012 study.[17]

When the tabulations were begun, the average age of all patients was about 54 years old but spanned a wide range of ages.[17] Patients who were prescribed sleeping pills tended to have more cases of disease at the outset than those not prescribed. No other disease besides insomnia was to be common amongst those receiving sleeping pills. There were other signs of stress in the prescribed group, for example, those not prescribed had about an 8% rate of being divorced whereas those prescribed had about a 12% rate.

Dr. Kripke and colleagues pointed out that as many as 15 smaller studies done before his large study reported similar results. In 2014, scientists in the UK conducted a similar study.[18] That study involved the healthcare records of 34,727 patients 16 or older years old who were first prescribed an anti-anxiety or hypnotic drug (94% of those were the long-acting benzodiazepines or the z-sleeping pills or both) and 69,418 patients (matched) with no prescriptions of those drugs. For each group there were records of the diagnosis for any presenting disease. The UK study's introduction cited research indicating that there was already documented evidence of adverse effects of using the drugs in question including the increased risk of dementia, problematic falls and accidents, cancer and pneumonia and other infections.

The results of the UK study can best be described by reporting the age of death. Those prescribed the benzodiazepines and Z-drugs (plus a few other drugs for anxiety and sleep problems) died at the average age of 76.2 years old, whereas those not so prescribed died at the average age of 82.1 years old (statistics indicate that this difference is highly unlikely to have occurred by chance). As with the Kripke et al.-study, both groups had patients that fall into various diagnoses; the difference being that more patients taking sleeping pills were diagnosed as having one of the previously mentioned diseases more than the controls. Given the most common causes of death, it is not surprising that 23.7% of those diagnosed with cancer were among the drug-users and 17.9% were among the nondrug-users; and 23.1% of users suffered from ischemic heart disease compared to 18.1% of nondrug-users.

Kripke continued to assess the risks in his 2016 article, "Hypnotic drug risks of mortality, infection, depression, and cancer: but lack of benefit" which was presented in October, 2015 to the Commissioner of the FDA and published in a peer-reviewed journal.[19] Kripke begins his review by pointing out that of the 40 research papers on mortality associated with hypnotics that 39 showed hypnotics were associated with excess death rates. He goes on to say "in 39 studies there was no evidence that hypnotics ever benefited patient survival."[19(p 2)]

Kripke explains why death due to hypnotics tends to occur at night. Hypnotics (which are agonists at the GABA receptors) facilitate neuronal inhibition; including the inhibition of centers in the brain that regulate breathing. This causes respiratory depression, i.e., breathing slowly diminishes until the individual just stops breathing. Alcohol and opioids (e.g., oxycodone) intake can also induce respiratory depression. Taking alcohol or opioids along with sleeping pills increases the risk of death from respiratory depression.

In his 2016 review, Kripke pointed out that a meta-analysis of hypnotics and infections clearly linked hypnotic-use with potentially serious infections, even those infections that are a leading cause of death (diseases of the lungs, such a pneumonia).[20] He goes on to point out that the relationship between hypnotic drugging and infection has been shown in animal studies which confirm a direct causal relationship between the drugs' actions and the development of serious infection.

Given these results, the American Geriatrics Society recommended in their 2015 report on potentially inappropriate medication-use in older adults that practitioners avoid prescribing benzodiazepines as anti-anxiety agents or as hypnotics to older citizens.[14] They graded all of their recommendations as either weak or strong and indicated that their recommendation to avoid these drugs as *strong* and the quality of the evidence as *high*. The American College of Physicians advised that hypnotics not be the first choice of therapy for insomnia and instead recommended cognitive behavioral therapy for insomnia (a process we will discuss later).

The American Academy of Sleep Medicine published revised clinical practice guidelines for the pharmacological treatments of chronic insomnia, for adults, in February 2017. They recommended 8 available medicines for treatment of sleep disorders that practitioners might consider prescribing and 6 not recommended, 4 of which are OTC drugs (diphenhydramine, melatonin, L-tryptophan and Valerian). They judged all their recommendations of medicines to be weak based primarily on the grounds that there was not sufficient available evidence. In their narrative, they acknowledged that cognitive behavioral therapy might be the superior first line approach to treating sleep disorders. This clinical practice guideline seems to be at odds with the data Kripke reviewed in as much as they recommended the Z-drugs and temazepam for clinical use whereas the Kripke-epidemiological data indicated that these drugs were associated with premature death and provided no benefit.

In Kripke's latest review, he extrapolated that recently as many as 300,000 to 500,000 premature deaths, per year, occur as a result of hypnotics and anti-anxiety drugs. Many of these drugs act as GABA agonists (enhance inhibition of neurons) or are anti-histaminergic drugs with an anticholinergic burden, that is, they interfere with the innate immune system of the airway and good thinking. *Given the mortality data, it is hard to recommend any available drug for insomnia.*

When you "screw around" with nearly all neurons of your brain; What do you suppose would be the consequences of that? Maybe, the result might be more car crashes, falls, poor decision-making, indulgence in unhealthy habits, poor impulse control and, now, we have also learned increased risks of infection and cancer. Maybe, just maybe, the accumulation of such might lead to an earlier death than if you had a safe alternative. There are safe alternatives and that is the focus for the rest of this book. However, we do discuss one more issue with drugs and health, polypharmacy.

Issues of Polypharmacy

Polypharmacy refers to the concurrent use of many drugs taken to treat diseases. It is not to be confused with addiction, the overuse of particular substances such as tobacco products, alcoholic beverages or pain-killers. Polypharmacy refers to the overuse of a variety of drugs typically prescribed by a doctor for the treatment of various ailments a person has. Polypharmacy leads to a host of negative side-effects. Often seniors that take sleeping pills take many other drugs to treat disease concurrently, thus endangering their health.

With age, the capability of our kidneys and liver to process medications slows down. This causes drugs to remain in blood longer thus increasing a drug's activity. This is further compounded by the fact that drugs can be stored in body fat and most people gain fat as they age. Since older individuals also tend to take more drugs, the likelihood for serious side-effects are elevated.

Prior to the Food and Drug Act of 1906, no Federal regulations (USA) controlled the sale of drugs and herbs that might be medicines. We use the term "might be" advisedly because what was sold was often not effective or was adulterated. Among the most common drugs sold by traveling salesmen was laudanum, a combination of opium and alcohol. Since that time, advances in knowledge of public health and biology have increased the life-span of citizens in prosperous nations. Since 1906, there have been major advances in the development and marketing of drugs.

Among the technical developments that have emerged since 1906 is the science of advertising and marketing whose findings are used by companies selling drugs. This science of marketing is manifest by the fact that universities can offer doctoral training programs in marketing and public relations. Currently, the advanced technology of sales (to produce ads and public relations) is purchased, at a yearly cost, of more than 5 billion dollars to promote the sale of drugs. These companies spend that money to increase sales and profits.

From 1906 until now, there has been a constant attempt by governmental regulations to provide useful, needed information, and to regulate the development, manufacture and sale of drugs in the service of providing safeguards for the population. The Federal agency with this responsibility is the FDA. The FDA is charged with the mandates drafted by the Congress of the USA and upheld by the executive and judicial branches of the Federal government.

The basic reason for the constant need to regulate the manufacture and sale of drugs is the simple fact that drugs can be, and often are, very powerful. A small pill can either cure a major disease and hence prolong a happier life or be a lethal agent, a poison that can kill in a matter of minutes or can kill in a matter of decades when used consistently. It is a matter of grave concern when a life-saving drug is not made available to all citizens. It is of grave concern when a drug is marketed whose effects induce life-threatening changes. And with the rise of psychopharmacology, there are similar grave concerns about drugs affecting how we think and feel.

The 4th leading cause of death in the USA is accidents and that includes death due to misuse of drugs (a vast majority of "accidents").

The modern drug market is composed of (a) prescription drugs authorized for use by a licensed professionals, usually a physician, (b) drugs sold "over-the-counter" (OTC) drugs which can be purchased without a prescription and are available at retail outlets, and (c) dietary supplements often sold in stores specializing in these products including vitamins and (d) illegal drugs which are often addictive substances that are outlawed by Federal and State Laws.

The rationale for limiting some drugs to be used only with the advice of some medical professionals (usually a physician with an M.D. or D.O. degree from a recognized medical college and licensed by the state in which the prescribing physician practices). That is, these drugs can be, if misused, disease-producing and in some cases lethal. Physicians are well-aware, by virtue of their extended, rigorous education and by their continued post-licensing self-directed education of the scientific basis for using a drug as a treatment for a disease.

Prescription Drugs

We looked for the number of prescription drugs that the FDA has approved. It was weird that the FDA did not have the number readily available. Other researchers who faced the same problem did the work to figure out that the number of drugs approved from 1827 to 2013 was 1453.[21] Some of these drugs have subsequently been declared as OTC drugs.

It is safe to say that physicians of the USA have a list of over 1400 FDA-approved drugs available to them to prescribe for their patients.

It is also safe to say that physicians do not prescribe that many drugs and none of them scan the full list of drugs to decide which of them to prescribe to any given patient. Even if they wished to prescribe a drug on that list, that drug may not be available at the local drug store. So, in the day-to-day practice of medicine only a relatively small number (which may be 20 or so, but never thousands) of drugs are available for the treatment of any given diagnosis. And, also relevant, there are more brands of drugs than active ingredients approved for treatment of a given diagnosis.

So, how does a physician make the decision to prescribe a drug to any given patient? Surely, the first step toward making the decision involves a diagnosis. For example, a patient might say that they have a problem with insomnia and then that becomes a diagnosis indicating that an FDA-approved, prescription hypnotic is called for. Most physicians are aware of commonly used sleep-aids. Further, in today's medical practice, a physician with his laptop can call up a list of sleep-aids with notes on how they work and their side-effects (but probably not their anticholinergic burden, discussed later). That information might include warnings posted by the FDA or occasionally by the drug-company as to serious and common problems associated with any particular drug.

Since only a licensed medical professional can write a prescription for FDA approved drugs, the pharmaceutical companies have sales representatives that visit those who can write prescriptions. It is unethical and illegal for licensed prescribers (e.g., doctors) to receive money or favors of any kind for prescribing a drug. This is an obvious understanding: A doctor should always make unbiased decisions about the health of a patient and the rule for preventing biased decisions is to decline any compensation for prescribing a drug.

The role of the pharmaceutical representatives is to "educate" the prescriber of the advantages of a drug being marketed by a company. They can do that, supposedly ethically, by conducting that education on a golf course or a cruise ship or at a nice restaurant, or at a convention in a nice city where there is a seminar educating on the latest medicines for which the drug-company pays all costs of the "educational experience." In other words, the drug-companies can provide favors under the guise of "education serving the prescribers," but, in fact, merely provide a sales-pitch designed to have the prescriber to prescribe the companies' drug. Really, it does not take a Ph.D. in marketing or psychology to know that people are more likely to incorporate your message if the message is given along with nice experiences that might, indeed, be costly but given freely, along with compliments for all your good work. In the modern scheme of things, it is likely that your doctor has an unwarranted bias toward certain drugs.

Most nations of the world, except the USA and New Zealand, either severely limit or do not permit the advertising of drugs, particularly prescription drugs. Many nations also dispel the false claims that are made by those selling prescription, OTC drugs and dietary supplements.

The allowed ads in the USA are regulated. For example, the ads for prescription drugs must report the common side-effects of the drugs and must advise viewers to consult your doctor (which is actually guidance on how to buy a prescription drug). The regulations for OTC and dietary supplements also must limit their claims and recommend that viewers seek professional medical advice before taking them (an act seldom taken).

OTC Drugs

Local drugstores can offer over 300,000 OTC drugs (brands) for sale. These brands contain upwards of 1000 active ingredients used in various combinations for the treatment of over 80 therapeutic classes of drugs. One of those categories is sleep-aids.[22]

The FDA decides which drugs may be approved for sale without a prescription. OTC-drugs are approved on the basis that these drugs are generally safe when used as directed by the information provided on the package-label or package-insert.

OTC drugs are not likely to be toxic when used as directed and temporarily. However, when used chronically, and in combination with other drugs, they can induce disease with even fatal consequences. We mentioned already, that adverse drug reactions account for a large proportion of accidental deaths in the United States which are now in the class labelled as unintended consequences, the fourth leading cause of death.[23] OTC drugs are often one of the combination of drugs producing the deadly consequences.

The ready availability, typically low cost (in comparison to prescription drugs) and the marketing associated with OTC products account for their widespread use. For example, the typical American consumer makes about 26 trips a year to a store to purchase OTC products. Further, each household spends about $338 a year on OTC products. The total OTC market is over $23 billion dollars.[24] Presumably, this self-medication saves total healthcare cost such as might be incurred by Medicaid and Medicare for visits to a doctor. However, if polydrug use leads to serious illnesses; obviously, then, there are no savings in overall healthcare costs.

The Dietary Supplement Market

In 1994, the US Congress passed a law indicating that a class of drugs were to be handled differently from other drugs, particularly different than many OTC drugs. This new class was to include nutraceuticals, botanicals, and food supplements (including vitamins). The law stipulated that these kinds of "drugs" could be marketed without premarket clearance by the FDA.[25] Consequently, now many so-called natural drugs are not screened for safety (and dosing) as are new OTC and prescription drugs.

The dietary supplement market (sometimes called the alternative medicine market) is not totally free of governmental regulation. For example, dietary supplements cannot claim to prevent, treat or cure disorders. However, they can say that the products have beneficial physical or psychological effects without having to prove those claims.

These products can be sold without clear labeling of what is supposed to be the active ingredient. They also don't need to provide information about safe-dosing or potential adverse effects. Unlike OTC drugs and prescription drugs, the FDA can only ban a supplement from the market if it is proven to be dangerous. Consequently, unsafe supplements can be freely sold until the FDA has done enough research to provide proof, beyond reasonable doubt, that a product presents a significant risk. A germane note: the staff of the FDA are overworked.

Also, dietary supplements do not have to list adverse effects. Please note that not all so called "natural" products are good for you. You should let your healthcare provider know if you are taking dietary supplements. Most suggest that these drugs should be counted as one of the five drugs used to define polypharmacy including the commonly known dietary supplements as a single pill of multiple vitamins.

The dietary supplements are recognized by the required label on their packages that "… has not been evaluated by the Food and Drug Administration" and "This product is not intended to diagnose, treat, cure or prevent any disease." Only a few dietary supplements have been investigated by the FDA for unsafe side effects. This happens only after they are already on the market. Please note that the dietary supplement "Kava root" is listed by the FDA as being toxic to the liver.[26] Also, please note, it is being advertised as a sleep-aid.

When citizens use the OTC market and the dietary supplement market, they are tasked to correctly diagnose their ailment, select the appropriate drug, and take the appropriate dose for the required length of time. To be safe, they must administer the drug as directed and store it properly for subsequent re-use. Many citizens do this, without any formal education in medicine, dentistry, veterinary medicine, nursing or pharmacology. Many parents do this for their children without the detailed knowledge of how to do so. Now, this would not be particularly problematic, if all these self-prescribed medicines were safe. *They are not all safe.* They are not all safe particularly when used in combination with other drugs.

The FDA recommends that one should receive advice on the safety of these dietary supplements from governmental sources rather than the manufacturers' advertisements.[26] This is the case because the advertisements and other kinds of marketing are often exaggerations of the benefits and overlook potential hazards (in other words, the ad-campaigns for many of this kind of product are sophisticated falsehoods). Citizens should watch out for comments like "These supplements are safe, natural, or have been used for centuries safely," and other exaggerations.

Most advertised advantages of these supplements have not been tested. Claims are often inconclusive or just plain lies. In fact, this is an extraordinarily, loosely regulated drug-market that is heavily advertised and marketed.

A goodly number of drugs can interact, in multiple ways, with one or more drugs (including dietary supplements) to produce serious adverse effects. Please note: Each dietary supplement and alternative medicine counts toward the number of drugs you are taking when assessing polypharmacy.

In one study, risk of an older adults experiencing a fall within 30 days after the prescription-drug has reached the patient increased by 7% for each additional medication taken.[27] Given the serious consequences of a fall among the older citizens, this becomes an additional, serious side-effect of polypharmacy.[23]

Unfortunately, since many physicians earn considerable money by prescribing drugs, it is not in their financial interests to curb drug-prescriptions. Of course, number of drugs sold, in turn, makes money for the pharmaceutical industry. Also, those who sell OTC drugs and dietary supplements have a vested interest in selling as many drugs as they can. All of this is aided and abetted by clever marketing (a money-making activity). All of the incentives seem to favor the selling of drugs. The result, all too often, is that polypharmacy is disease-producing rather than healing.

Citizens of the USA pay more for each of the drugs they use than any other nation. Also, the total healthcare budget, per citizen, is greater in the USA than other nations in part due to the treatment of drug-overdoses. If you are taking five or more drugs, it is time to ask your healthcare provider to select the few drugs that are best for you and stop taking too many drugs.

Data from the CDC indicates that for all ages, both sexes, the percent of the USA population that took five or more prescription drugs in the 30 days prior to being asked about their drug-intake was, on average, 10.9%. For males aged 65 years of more the percent was

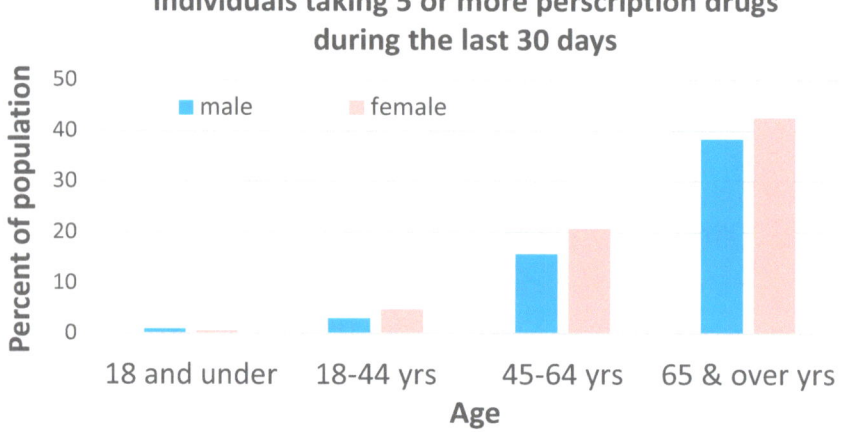

38.4; for females aged 65 years or more the percent was 42.[28] The same source was used to plot the graph.

In addition to the intake of prescription drugs, it is likely that 47% of the population also take OTC medications, and 54% take a dietary supplement (probably mostly vitamins but also hormones). Some research suggests that as many as 59% of patients are taking one or more unnecessarily prescribed drug.

Approximately 40% of American nursing home patients take more than *nine drugs*.[27] In Canada, however, only about 16% of nursing home patients are taking more than nine drugs.[27] It is difficult to make the case that Canadian citizens are not receiving adequate medicines. However, the extreme use of drugs by the elderly in nursing homes makes a lot of money for drug-companies which is usually paid for by taxes. This is at best inefficient and at worse just wrong; unequivocally wrong.[28]

Hans Selye, the father of stress research, made the case some years ago that stress affected so many biological systems adversely that stress itself should be considered a disease needing to be treated. We believe, following the same logic, that *polypharmacy can adversely affect so many biological systems that polypharmacy should be considered a disease needing to be treated.*

We hold that it is almost certain that anyone taking nine or more drugs simultaneously, some of which may directly affect the brain, would have serious, *adverse disruptions* on the complex physiology of sleep. This must be the case because of the simple fact that sleep occupies at least a fifth to a third or more of our lives.

Furthermore, anyone taking many drugs will almost inevitably sustain enough of what is called the anticholinergic burden (to be discussed in the next section) to cause serious disruptions in sleep and increase the risk of Alzheimers.

The most serious outcome of polypharmacy is, of course, death. The latest data posted on the website of the Centers for Disease Control and Prevention (the CDC) on causes of death indicate that accidents (unintentional injuries) are the 4th leading cause of death and the clear majority of those are due to misuse of drugs.[23] Death associated with drugs is most often due to one or more drugs interacting inducing fatal disease, i.e., a function of polypharmacy. The 10th leading cause of death is suicide which is often due to voluntarily taking lethal doses of drugs.[23] We have more to say on the issue of drug-use and mortality, but now we address another issue associated with taking multiple drugs at the same time.

The Anticholinergic Burden

Rarely, does a drug work without producing at least some side-effects. While some of these side-effects are apparent upon taking the drug; others are not. If one takes many drugs chronically, as the millions of Americans affected by polypharmacy do, these negative effects can combine to produce drastic results.

One such side-effect is an anticholinergic effect which deals with the potential malfunctioning of the neurotransmitter, acetylcholine. Neurotransmitters are substances released by neurons. When they act on another neurons, they transmit information.

The brain uses as many as 200 different neurotransmitters to sustain its complicated actions, allowing us to behave efficiently as we adapt to changing circumstances. The disruption of any one of these neurotransmitters of the brain is apt to be problematic.

Acetylcholine is one of the more important neurotransmitters; because it is involved in multiple circuits of the brain and peripheral nervous system. Among these circuits are those associated with memory formation and memory recall. As you all know, loss of memory is a major symptom of Alzheimers.

Given the fact that anticholinergics are associated with cognitive decline, it would be prudent to know which drugs inhibit cholinergic activity; that is, have an anticholinergic burden. Often, there are other drugs for the same diagnosis that have little or no anticholinergic burden. Consequently, scientists compiled lists of drugs and their anticholinergic ratings. Many commonly used drugs have either a direct effect or a side-effect that is anticholinergic. If an individual takes, for example, two or three of these drugs, the combined anticholinergic effect will induce noticeable cognitive problems.

Doctors should consider the ramifications of any drugs they prescribe that have an anticholinergic burden, especially if the patient is taking multiple drugs. The scientific community has assessed the anticholinergic burden of a large number of the commonly used drugs and those findings are available to physicians and pharmacists.

Here we can provide this information. Many of the OTC and dietary supplement drugs advertised as sleep-aids and as medicines for the common cold have a considerable anticholinergic burden. Specifically, we advise older citizens to not use pills containing this antihistamine: diphenhydramine. In part, we advise this because diphenhydramine has a considerable anticholinergic burden in addition to inducing other problems.

We take this opportunity to tell you that the only medicines that have any positive effects associated with halting the cognitive decline of Alzheimer's disease is a cholinergic drug. These drugs effectively increase the acetylcholine in the brain thereby temporarily slowing down the process of cognitive decline. Unfortunately, these cholinergic drugs do not halt the progression of brain damage nor do they repair the damage already done. They provide a temporary fix that is eventually undone by the processes that are Alzheimers.

Managing Polypharmacy

You should take an inventory of the drugs you take regularly including all OTC and dietary supplements. The list should include agents often not considered to be drugs, but which are, such as alcoholic beverages and tobacco products. If the list is more than 5 drugs you and your doctor or pharmacist should determine which of the list can be eliminated without doing harm. This will prepare you for a time when you really need a medicine for a new disease affecting you. Your professional healthcare providers can also tabulate your anticholinergic burden due to multiple drug use. Also, your professional healthcare advisor should be aware of the Beers Criteria Medication report. The Beer's report is the American Geriatrics Society's list for potentially inappropriate medications for older adults.

Drug-Withdrawal

Depending on the drug you have been taking regularly, the withdrawal effects from taking that drug can vary from being very serious to a minor inconvenience. The severity and duration of withdrawal depends on the drug and your history of taking it. The greater the dose of a drug and the longer you have been taking it, the more severe the withdrawal.

Withdrawal from taking large amounts of alcoholic beverages and taking large amounts of opioid pain-killers (e.g., morphine or OxyContin) daily requires medical management. Withdrawal from extensive use of alcoholic beverages or pain-killers is not something you should try to manage by yourself. There are centers for managing that in nearly every large city usually associated with a local hospital. The best advice: Make an appointment at one of those centers, keep that appointment and understand you are apt to suffer some withdrawal, but you will gain a better life.

If you have been regularly taking a sleeping pill or antianxiety drug with benzodiazepine as the active ingredient, and you stop taking that pill, it is highly likely you will experience some withdrawal symptoms. The withdrawal symptoms are likely to be insomnia and anxiety. Note: After habitually taking the pills you might experience some benefit just after taking them, but you will most likely experience being (a) groggy and tired the day afterwards, (b) some hindrance in memory processing and (c) further insomnia and anxiety when you stop taking them.

For dealing with chronic insomnia, CBT-I works better and has none of the drawbacks listed above. Further, CBT-I does not put you at risk for polypharmacy and anticholinergic burden. Even further, you can probably manage CBT-I by yourself. If self-managed CBT-I helps only very little (an unlikely possibility if engaged), you surely retain the option of seeking professional help. The results of extensive research support the conclusion that CBT-I can be managed by individuals with some instruction and some motivation to try those practices.

Consider these understandings: Sleeping pills should not be used regularly. They have only been approved by the FDA for temporary use. Hypnotics have some addictive potential which often leads to them being taken regularly even when that is not recommended. However, they do provide some sense of satisfaction immediately after taking them. That experience might indicate that they are doing good. However, the longer-term effects can become serious problems. When you stop taking them, the withdrawal effects are insomnia and anxiety. Taking these sleeping pills for insomnia does induce the unconsciousness of the beginnings of sleep which *seems* O.K., but they also suppress REM-sleep (which you do not experience directly), which is *not* O.K. The net effect is inefficient sleep which is self-diagnosed as insomnia and a felt need for taking a sleeping pill. As you can clearly imagine, this can set a habit that is maladaptive; a vicious circle or an addiction.

Many drugs we (the population) take often and regularly induce noticeable withdrawal symptoms. As mentioned, alcoholic beverages and opioid pain-killers are notorious for severe withdrawal. However, other drugs also elicit withdrawal symptoms when use is stopped or significantly slowed down. Regular use of tobacco and marijuana products induce withdrawal when stopped. Antianxiety drugs as well as anti-depressants elicit withdrawal symptoms when their use is stopped. Coffee has mild but noticeable withdrawal effects usually manifest by headaches and irritability.

For those substances for which you can reduce the dose systematically, say use of alcoholic beverages, the advice is to taper use gradually, systematically and regularly to avoid severe withdrawal effects. It helps to do this regularly and systematically by keeping a record of your intake. It is often very difficult or impossible to systematically to reduce the dose of some drugs because pills come in only a few doses.

It is useful to understand that acute withdrawal symptoms usually last for only a matter of days. Craving for the highly addictive drugs, however, is often very persistent and can be felt even years after stopping the intake of these drugs.

Also, chronic intake often leads to tolerance, i.e., the drugs do not work as well at what was desired and often achieved with initial dosing. So, the net effect is little of what was desired and an increasing risk of adversity when stopped.

No matter what the drug, whether a prescription drug, an OTC drug or a nutritional supplement, the sellers have a vested interest in having you take the drug chronically and even for the rest of your life. That may not be in your best interest.

Commerce Associated with Sleeping

The large commercial interests associated with sleeping can and do work toward shaping our behavior to buy sleep-related products. In their quest to make profits, companies have developed highly sophisticated ways of influencing our thinking and our behavior about sleep. To fully understand sleep in our modern world, we need to also understand how modern commerce affects our sleep.

In a following section, we'll look at how commercial interests can affect the commerce of selling drugs and affect regulatory issues. Here, we mention that there are other commercial interests associated with sleep.

For example, the global market in 2017 for mattress-sales alone was worth US$27.87 billion and is expected to grow at a steady rate to reach US$43.43 billion by the end of 2024.[29] There are large markets in sheets, pillows, bedspreads and bedroom clothes.

The bedding-market like other markets is dynamic with a variety of new products being offered as well as new marketing schemes such as shopping via the internet. New companies are challenging the industry leaders. In addition to the bedding market and the drug-market there is an emerging market in devices that can monitor sleep as well as vital signs such as heart rate.

Vested Interests

We include three "case histories" on how governmental-commercial interactions can be a major factor in how an individual might deal with their sleep or their pain. We do this because understanding a bit of history can allow one to critically re-examine platitudes such as "medicines are good." If you are looking for quick advice on how to deal with your insomnia, skip to the Cognitive Behavioral Therapy for Insomnia.

At the Law-Making Level

Our current laws allow dietary supplements and anabolic steroids to be sold without any prior approval from the FDA. The fact that such gross lapses of oversight exist should invite skepticism on the part of consumers. Some sleep aids are dietary supplements and do have serious adverse effects which only were published by the FDA after they had already been on the market. Understanding a bit of the historical context can help explain how decisions at the law-making level affect the drugs that are available to consumers.

The Dietary Supplement Health and Education Act of 1994 (DSHEA) allowed dietary supplements to be sold without prior screening by the FDA for negative health effects.[25] The Law was introduced by Orrin Hatch (Republican Senator from Utah) and Tom Harken (Democratic Senator from Iowa) and signed into law by Pres. Bill Clinton, a Democrat. There seems to be a consensus that without the advocacy of Senator Hatch, the bill would not have been passed. Throughout his tenure as a Senator (to retire in 2018) Senator Hatch has been a strong defender of the law he championed and has thwarted attempts to correct what many thought to be the law's deficiencies. Needless to say: The bill clearly favored the dietary supplement industry and alternative medicine advocates. Those interests lobbied vigorously for the bill's passage.

Since the passage of the 1994 bill, the American supplement industry has grown into a market worth over $30 billion.[30] Increases in this market are fueled by extensive advertisements extolling the virtues of natural medicines and criticizing their better regulated pharmaceutical counterparts.

From 1989 to 1994, Senator Hatch received as much as $169,300 from companies selling herbal medicines and other dietary supplements. His former law partner began a dietary supplement company, based in Utah, Pharmics. In 2003, it was reported that Senator Hatch owned 35,621 shares in the company.

The Senator's son, Scott Hatch, has been a registered lobbyist and a partner in a law firm, Walker, Martin & *Hatch*, LLC. The main trade association for the pharmaceutical industry has as its short name PhRMA. PhRMA paid Walker, Martin & *Hatch*, in 2007,

$120,000 to lobby Congress on pending FDA regulations.

In response to athletes' use of newly developed hormonal substances to increase muscle strength and particularly relevant to Olympic competition, the Congress of the USA passed a new law to control the sale and distribution of these new drugs mimicking hormones. The full title of this Law is "The Designer Anabolic Steroid Control Act of 2014 to amend the Controlled Substance Act to more effectively regulate anabolic steroids." This law effectively outlaws newly developed anabolic steroids that might be used to enhance athletic performance.

However, the Law also defines hormonal substances that are not to be regulated as prescription drugs and, therefore, allowing them to be sold as nutritional substances. The law explicitly defines anabolic steroids as products that might enhance testosterone production *except* "estrogen, progesterone, corticosteroids and dehydroepiandrosterone" (the last of the list is known as DHEA). DHEA is the hormonal precursor of testosterone and estrogen. The effect of the Law is to make DHEA a nutritional supplement sold in the vitamin section of your local drug store.

Scott Hatch was a paid lobbyist for the nutritional substance trade association making it possible for the nearly unregulated sale of drugs that enhance hormonal production for whatever purported use that can be advertised, e.g., muscle building and enhanced sexuality. Of course, Senator Hatch had no role in promoting a voice vote for the senate passage of the bill despite his long-term advocacy of the nutritional supplement industry. However, his son did receive compensation for lobbying for the bill to enhance the product line of the nutritional supplement industry and, in so doing reduce the regulatory oversight of the FDA.

Senator Hatch, his family and friends profited from the Senator's law-making opportunities. This unethical conduct, manifest as a clear conflict of interests, has been exposed several times. For example, his home town newspaper *The Salt Lake Tribune* stated in an editorial that Senator Hatch has an "utter lack of integrity." In 2011, the New York Times ran an article describing how a powerful senior senator (Hatch) became active in supporting pharmaceutical concerns raising his chances of increasing both his and his friend's wealth.[31] The Senator will retire in 2018 with a slightly tarnished reputation, but a considerably richer man who has helped his family become wealthy by promoting legislation that is in his personal interests. We take this excursion into the Law-making regulating the drug markets to warn you that decisions made with respect to the regulation of drugs in the USA may not be in your best interests.

At the Drug-Company Level

This subsection traces, briefly, the development and discovery of the first effective drug to be used as a medicine. It also looks at how the drug company's use of all the technics of modern medical chemistry and modern marketing led to a monumental disaster, i.e., we discuss the modern opioid crises.

The ancients discovered that a product of the poppy plant (now called opium) was useful in controlling diarrhea, coughing and, of great value in controlling pain. They also knew that it could induce something resembling sleep. They also discovered that it induced a pleasurable state.

73

The ancients cultivated the poppy plant (one of the first adventures in agriculture along with the cultivation of wheat) and over centuries considerable commerce centered around opium. The availability of opium provided the first real medicines for controlling some fatal diseases; for example, uncontrolled diarrhea is fatal especially to babies and small children and the availability of opium was life-saving. For centuries, opium was used as medicine.

When opium was plentiful, it was also used to instill the pleasant state usually by way of inhaling the smoke of heated opium. Using opium to induce pleasure developed into a habit. The habit of taking opium leads to several unpleasant consequences. One of them is that smoking opium induces itching. Another is constipation. Also, tolerance develops so that to achieve any benefit from taking the drugs, more and more of it needs to be taken to achieve the benefit. Unfortunately, for the regular user, the tolerance develops sooner for actions such as pain-relief than for constipation. So, taking greater doses helps in controlling pain but exacerbates itching and constipation.

When a habit of using is stopped, there are withdrawal effects. The withdrawal effects were nearly the opposite of what the drug induced and one of which is diarrhea and stomach pains, i.e., the functional equivalent of disease. The medicine to prevent withdrawal is to take more opium inducing the dual effect of some pleasure and relief of disease. So, the phenomena of an intense addiction became part of human culture characterized by the addict (a new word was added to our lexicon) willing to spend a great deal of time and resources on acquiring opium.

There was commerce associate with opium as a medicine and as an addictive agent. This made the cultivation of the poppy plant and the refinement of the product of that plant, a large worldwide enterprise. Among the most successful of that commercial enterprises was the British East India Company (a private company begun in 1600 by Queen Elizabeth I which held a monopoly on trade between Britain and India to 1858). This trade stoked considerable wealth for Britain and its world-wide colonies. Among their most profitable commodities was trade in opium.

At the dawn of the 19th century, a young German scientist, Friedrich Sertürner, isolated the active ingredient in opium and named it morphine, for the Greek god of sleep, Morpheus. This act, in turn, began the medicinal chemistry that supports a great deal of the modern pharmaceutical world.

The medicinal chemistry associated with morphine was directed toward finding medicines for the various actions of morphine, i.e., anti-coughing, anti-diarrhea and better pain control that was not addicting or did not have the same constellation of effects as morphine. For example, a goal was to make drugs that might control coughing, and concurrently not be addictive or have side-effects such as constipation. That medicinal chemistry was remarkably successful and almost all modern cough medicines is a product of that chemistry. An active ingredient in almost all cough medicines is dextromethorphan hydrobromide and that is the active ingredient in one of the most popular brands of cough medicines, Robitussin.

The research directed toward finding a medicine that might control pain without being addicting failed. We now know a great deal about the behavioral neuroscience associated with pain and a great deal about how morphine can control pain. For example, morphine acts on specific receptors in the areas of the brain whose activity is experienced as pain and we know the genes that produce the proteins that make up those receptors. We know there are receptors in the gut for which morphine acts. That knowledge explains morphine's ability to produce constipation and the diarrhea associated with withdrawal from the near daily use of morphine.

A large field of poppy plants[32]

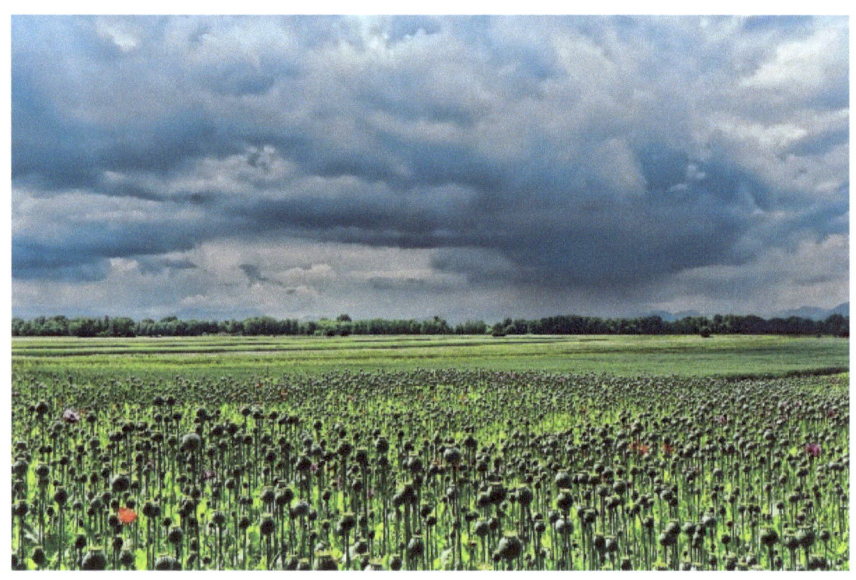

The medicinal chemists in coordination with physiologists (pharmacologists) have developed both new long-acting analgesic drugs as well as short-acting ones. Pharmaceutical companies have patented these drugs, have gained the right to market these drugs and have marketed them aggressively. These drugs, because of the potential to be addictive, are prescription drugs.

Among the long-acting drugs developed and marketed was oxycodone (brand name: OxyContin) marketed by *Purdue Pharma*. Hence begins one of the saddest episodes in the commercial history of the United States. In the United States, in 2016, there were 63,600 drug-overdose-deaths of which it is likely that 42,000 of those were directly related to the inhalation or injection of an opioid analgesic (pain controlling medicine). The latest data indicate that overdose-induced deaths have reached (circa 2017) 72,000 despite some efforts to improve the situation at the root of the problem. Over the course of the last 16 years, the numbers of deaths due to overdoses have risen dramatically, year by year. According to the CDC, the rate of death due to drug overdoses was five times higher in 2016 than in 1999. The cumulative effect of this circumstances has led to the death of over 200,000 citizens. Note: During that same 15 years, the USA has been at war. The cumulative death rate of all our wars during that same period is considerably less than 200,000.

Purdue Pharma pled guilty to misleading prescribers and users of the drug's risk of addiction. The only repercussions for Purdue Pharma were a series of fines which were of little consequence to the company and those that worked for it. Purdue pharma paid $600 million. The Purdue president paid $19 million. Purdue's top lawyer paid $8 million. Purdue's former medical director paid $7.5 million. For a company which made $2.8 billion in revenue from 1995-2001, this was surely not a big burden.

Purdue Pharma continues to sell drugs including OxyContin to this day. Further, they have expanded their sales to other countries using the same false advertising they used in the USA. Purdue Pharma's 2017 revenue was thought to be over 3 billion US dollars. Purdue Pharma is a private company whose false advertising and lack of ethical behavior has led to hundreds of thousands of deaths.

Generally, there is a consensus: morphine and similar opioids are very good at controlling acute pain due to such as broken legs or kidney stones. Unfortunately, those same drugs are not very effective for controlling chronic pain. The drug sold by Purdue Pharma was touted to be a drug to control chronic pain and if true would be a valuable drug. Unfortunately, data collected by others than Purdue Pharma indicate that it is not particularly effective in controlling chronic pain, but we have discovered it is highly addictive.

At the company level, there can be excessive greed and that greed, in turn, has led to the modern opioid crisis.

At the FDA Level

In a 2018 issue of the prestigious journal *Science*, an article was published exposing another way a vested interest can modify the drugs made available to you.[33]

Before a drug can be approved by the FDA, a panel of experts consisting of medical researchers and advisors gather to decide to approve or not to approve a drug for therapeutic use. Panel members study the available research and listen to presentations on results from preclinical and clinical trials from drug-makers and eventually vote on whether or not to approve of the drug.

The FDA has systems in place to identify possible conflicts of interest for each panel member. Surprisingly, reports are showing that some of the panel members received compensation from these companies in the form of money for travel, research, honoraria and consultations. These payments are made either before the drug approval panel meeting or in the subsequent months or even years after the panel members voted on a drug. An analysis of the total compensation paid to 61% of the 107 physicians who advised the FDA on 28 drugs approved from 2008 to 2014 showed that the amount received by each physician varied from $1,000 to more than $1million.

Some of approved-drugs can be fatal when mixed with other drugs, as is the case of Seroquel. Seroquel is an antipsychotic produced by AstraZeneca that is linked to sudden cardiac death. In 2011, a young soldier, Jacob Sitko, was taking a mixture of drugs including Seroquel to treat his posttraumatic stress disorder. As a consequence, he died at the young age of 21 even though he was apparently in good health, except for his stress disorder. Two years prior, two panels had gathered to approve the use of Seroquel to treat schizophrenia and bipolar disorder in children, and depression in adults taking other medicines. The drug was then known to cause sudden cardiac death when used with certain drugs, but the results from the company's clinical studies showed minimal risks. Both panels voted to approve Seroquel for use and in the years following, several members from the panels received substantial financial contributions from AstraZeneca and the makers of competing drugs. Records from 2013 to 2016 showed that one of the FDA advisors who sat on one of the two panels had received $63,000 from AstraZeneca and $1.3 million from competitors.

These "pay later" conflicts of interest have largely gone unnoticed despite efforts by the FDA to identify and remove possible conflicts of interest for all voting panelists. The main reason being that the safeguards put in place by the FDA are not designed to prevent future monetary ties. In addition, some of the conflicts may be in the form of financial support from the drug-maker or key competitors for consulting on research which may be harder to track otherwise. Some panelists are more likely to vote for the approval of a drug if there is a possibility that there will be a future benefit from having a positive relationship with the company. These benefits are abundant and could be in the form of career advancement, compensation, research funding, or professional prestige and influence.

Apparently, it is common knowledge that if reviewers vote to approve a drug, then they are likely to gain from that action. Hence, the possibility of a biased decision.

The drugs approved by the FDA are not always free from partiality based on undisclosed conflicts of interest benefiting some of the members who sit on panels to approve these drugs.

Integrated Cognitive Behavioral Therapy (CBT) for Alzheimers

One of us (Larry) is a co-author of a major scientific review which concluded that Biologically Informed Cognitive Behavioral Therapy (CBT) is the optimal way of preventing Alzheimers. The goal of this therapy is to change maladaptive beliefs and behaviors and encourage adaptive beliefs and behaviors such that a person will take necessary *actions* to prevent Alzheimers.

Repeated behaviors often establish habits, and habits guide most ongoing behaviors. We can execute certain habitual tasks almost unconsciously, almost instinctually. A well-executed habit is a product of changes in the anatomy and physiology of one's brain, thereby allowing behavior to become more efficient at executing the engrained habit. This rather new understanding has a name; *brain plasticity*.

Brain plasticity is somewhat different than ordinary learning, (e.g., the learning of the names of capitals of the states of the USA). The *brain-plasticity-effect* involves a change in the organization of the brain, modifying both anatomy and physiology. While not readily apparent, these changes can be observed when taking detailed measurements.

If what we *do* modifies what we *are,* that opens *the possibility to use behavioral technologies to modify our physiology to become what we wish to be.* From the perspective of this book, as part of The Alzheimers Prevention Project, we presume that all of us would rather have a healthy brain as we age rather than one slowly descending into dementia. To fulfill that desire, we can attend to what we do. Since what we believe affects what we do, the cognitive part of this therapy involves assessing our beliefs to determine whether they are adaptive or not. This optimistic approach stands in stark contrast to the negative belief that there is no way you can prevent Alzheimer's disease and one can only wait for a medicine to cure the disease.

There are surely limits to what we can do to change ourselves. However, we now understand the scope of change that is possible is much greater than previously believed. The understanding that repeated behaviors can produce fundamental changes in the brain also has the implication that we have some control over the functionality of the brain. The contrasting idea is that brains become fixed during maturation and, therefore, we are left with few ways of changing our brain. Research indicates that brain plasticity can extend to even the oldest old ages.

Here, we are focused on habits associated with sleeping. Developed habits can sustain healthy sleep. Other developed habits can hinder healthy sleep. Healthy sleep, in turn, sustains the health of the brain. A healthy brain, in turn, helps us to continually shape our habitual behavior for maximum adaptability.

Of course, disease can be caused by toxins, infections, accidents, and by behaviors that increase the possibility for these insults. Note, however, by making certain choices and avoiding others, we can minimize our exposure to toxins, infections and reduce accidents. And, if we have the misfortune to become diseased resulting from a variety of circumstances, as a citizen of the modern world, we have opportunities to engage in practices that can restore our health.

The conceptualization of a biologically informed CBT may not be sufficiently broad to address the circumstances affecting the prevention of Alzheimers. We are going to use the next few pages to demonstrate how we must consider the circumstances in which we live to have a full understanding of how to be healthy. We now hold that biologically informed CBTs for prevention of Alzheimers should be broadened to a *biologically and sociologically informed cognitive behavioral technologies (CBTs) for Alzheimers*. We hoped to have made this modification clear by discussing the commercial circumstances associated with polypharmacy and the influence of vested interests that affect the regulation of the drug-market.

This book was designed to inform you about how to address a major risk for developing Alzheimer's disease, i.e., insomnia. Our approach considers biological and sociological circumstances (including our commercial culture) while addressing the risks incurred by insomnia. This is an integrated way of addressing issues of sleep problems which, in turn, addresses a risk for developing Alzheimers.

So, let us begin by learning about how to manage insomnia in our modern culture and develop behavioral and cognitive practices that will most likely ensure a good night's sleep.

Cognitive Behavioral Technologies for Insomnia (CBTs-I)

The scientific literature on cognitive behavioral practices for insomnia used this label: Cognitive Behavioral Therapy for Insomnia, CBT-I. We question the use of therapy in the title for nonpharmacological ways of managing problems of aging. Therapy implies a rather narrow range of interactions between a care-giver and a patient.

In a few pages from now, we are going to advise many individuals suffering insomnia to redecorate their bedrooms as one way, along with other ways, to achieve a goal of overcoming chronic insomnia. Redecorating a room can be therapeutic, but it is not really therapy, it is merely a known practice that research has indicated might be helpful. It is a technic, an action, not necessarily guided by a professional healthcare provider. You can change the physical appearance of your bedroom without receiving a bill for advice to do so and without being subject to a co-pay. To accommodate the broader perspective on the kinds of actions you can take to manage insomnia, we will use this title: cognitive behavioral technologies for insomnia or CBTs-I. This is part of a larger program of cognitive behavioral technologies for the prevention of Alzheimer's disease or CBTs-AD.

Along the lines advocating for a more integrative and proven approach to overcoming insomnia, we advocate only practices to overcome insomnia that are based in a scientific understanding of the biology and sociology inherent to the problem.

Science on Biologically and Sociological Informed CBTs-I

In 1999, the scientific journal *Sleep,* featured an article reviewing the evidence regarding the efficacy of nonpharmacological treatments for chronic insomnia.[34] The review was associated with the American Academy of Sleep Medicine, an organization primarily for physicians who specialize in treating sleep disorders such as sleep apnea and who manage sleep centers of the broader healthcare system. The 1999-review studied 48 clinical trials in which treatments for insomnia were assessed. The article's conclusion can be summarized by this statement: 70 to 80% of patients treated with technics now used in modern CBT-I benefited from the treatment. Based on the findings, practice guidelines were devised for day to day interactions with patients.[35]

After the 1999 article, more clinical trials and reviews of those trials further bolstered the idea that CBT-I was the preferred method for treating insomnia. One such review occurred in 2009[36] and others occurred in more recent years.[37,38] The research consistently supports the conclusion that CBT-I is effective. These findings have been endorsed by organizations representing the medical professions such as the American College of Physicians.[39]

Unfortunately, the USA's current healthcare system has incentivized pharmacological treatments over CBTs-I. Consequently, citizens presenting with insomnia are still being treated in large numbers by prescription hypnotics, OTC drugs and dietary supplements.[40] Large numbers of citizens are not being treated by CBTs-I which is the preferred, proven treatment that is not only effective, but a safe alternative.

Fortunately, citizens have the ability to do for themselves what they need to do to achieve healthy sleep. That is: They can learn how to engage CBTs-I and then practice that learning and develop the habits that will sustain healthy sleep. This book has been designed to educate you in the technics of CBTs-I and help you to engage them. If you engage CBTs-I you will reduce the risk of developing Alzheimer's disease as well as other diseases.

Fundamentals of CBTs-I

We now fully understand that our brains are molded by what we do; and then that molded brain guides what we do. This unending circle (unending reciprocity) continues even into old age. An implication of this modern understanding is: *By behaving consistently in a prescribed way, one can induce the changes in the brain to sustain a routine of healthy sleep.*

Also, how we behave tends to determine how we think. Ongoing behavior interacts with our unique human brain to develop concepts (beliefs, attitudes, construals) helpful in guiding behavior.

Fortunately, as well as unfortunately, beliefs and well-established habits tend not to be easily modified. If engrained habits changed easily and momentarily, they would, in fact, not be useful. On the other hand, if beliefs are not in accordance with reality, their persistence in guiding behavior is a problem.

Our education often establishes enduring, useful beliefs which become stronger as we act on them. For example, it is common to believe that brushing your teeth morning and evening is a good, useful habit. Now, if someone told you brushing that often is not healthy and you should brush only once a week, you would undoubtedly question that advice. Your belief in at-least-twice-daily-brushing has been told to you by your parents, teachers, dentists and millions of ads encouraging buying toothpaste and toothbrushes. So, you believe the advice, you sustain the habit and buy dental supplies. Generally, daily dental care is in concordance with our beliefs and is highly adaptive and even further presents no conflicts that might produce uneasiness. There are beliefs about sleep that are as engrained as your belief in brushing your teeth daily but may not be as adaptive. If a belief about sleep turns out to be maladaptive, then it would be rational to develop a contrary belief.

What changes bad habits? The answer is developing new good habits. Insomnia is often the result of bad habits and maladaptive beliefs. CBTs-I is the development of good habits and adaptive beliefs about sleep. Replacing maladaptive habits with adaptive ones takes some effort and weeks of activity. If you have the means to understand most of the contents of this book, you can engage CBTs-I and regularly achieve healthy sleep.

The goal of CBTs-I is to encourage beliefs that are concordant with adaptive behavior thereby sustaining the daily habit of healthy sleep which, in turn, is conducive to overall health and longevity.

Although we each and all have had the experience of living daily with day turning into night and night turning into day, we may have our own well-established beliefs about sleep and sleeping. These beliefs are supported by our experiences and by our education on sleep from various sources. As mentioned in the first part of this book, there are significant commercial interests in sleep-products including, of course, the drugs prescribed and advertised to treat insomnia. These commercial enterprises have vested interests in instilling certain beliefs in potential customers. We will explore some of those beliefs as we discuss some of the cognitive features of CBTs-I.

A Noteworthy Feature of CBTs-I

There is a fundamental difference between CBTs-I and being prescribed a drug to correct chronic insomnia. Taking drugs is a rather passive act, as one expects the drug to do "the work" of correcting the insomnia. In contrast, CBT-I requires thinking and then mobilizing behaviors to correct any identified problem.

When citizens take charge of their treatment by actively following the procedures of CBTs-I, they are likely to improve their sleep quality. This book is designed to provide you some help, so you can manage *your* treatment of *your* insomnia. Fortunately, the amount of work to change *your* thinking and behavior in the service of better sleep is not difficult but does need some attention. It will take some time. If done well, healthy sleep habits eventually become nearly instinctual.

When individuals take charge of their insomnia-treatment, research confirms that self-help-CBTs-I is effective. Research indicates that there is little difference between CBTs-I delivered over the internet and direct face to face interaction with a therapist. They both provide education and encouragement.[41]

Both CBTs-I via Internet and CBTs-I via reading a book (bibliotherapy) provide some expert advice. When that advice gets translated into active behavior, there is a strong likelihood of a reduction of insomnia and the establishment of a healthy pattern of sleep. A beneficial side-effect of CBTs-I via the internet or via a relevant book is that both are available without leaving the comfort of your home and are inexpensive compared to face to face professional advice. Further, there are many places in the USA where there are no professionals focusing on sleep. However, the internet and books are widely accessible.

CBTs-I, regardless of how they are engaged, are remarkably straightforward. CBTs-I involve changing bad habits into good ones and replacing maladaptive beliefs with adaptive ones. The formation of any habit, even bad ones, takes practice. Consistent practice can lead to good habits. It is essential, therefore, to take the time and effort to engage sustained practice in the service of adaptive habits.

There is Value to Regular Medical Checkups

Before we start a discussion of CBTs-I, please, understand that there are serious diseases that have the effect of inducing insomnia. Some examples are acid reflux, sleep apnea or arthritic pain. Therefore, it is good advice to see your healthcare professional for regular physical check-ups to detect any disease before it becomes truly troubling. During that check-up, please tell your doctor about any problems you may have, particularly those involving blockage of the airway.

CBTs-I

We now begin considering cognitions and activities that will establish habits that will greatly reduce your risk of insomnia. Some of those activities can and should be done during your awake time; not during the time for sleep.

The next segment of this book follows a pattern. We ask some questions, you answer those questions as best you can and then there is a discussion of the answers. After the discussion of the answers, there is advice on how to manage your sleep. The result is a rather straightforward way of tailoring your CBTs-I to be suitable for you.

Question

I. Which of the following are the *necessary* hours of sleep to be healthy?

    a. 8 hours
    b. 7.5 hours
    c. 7 hours
    d. None of the above

Answer

The best answer to the above question is *None of the above*. There was a time when it was common knowledge that 8 hours of sleep was optimal (even necessary) for health and well-being. The CDC (USA's Centers for Disease Control and Prevention) now has as a "correct" answer 7 hours and make the claim that anything less than 7 hours of sleep a day is not healthy. The optimal hours of sleep during a 24-hour period to be healthy depends on a number of factors and there is no one correct answer.

Consultation

There is no controversy: Sleep is necessary. However, there is some debate over how much sleep is necessary to sustain optimal health. Distinguished scientists who have devoted considerable time to the study of sleep and health-related issues differ in their estimates of how much sleep one needs. Several estimates for the sleep-time *necessary* for an adult's optimal health is *at least* 5.75, 6.5, 7.0 or 8.0 hours of sleep-time. Babies, young children, adolescents and those in the 6th to 9th decades of life vary from these numbers. Generally, younger individuals need more sleep while older ones require less.

The question is asked: How many hours of sleep are *necessary* for optimal health? Those asking the question wish for a concrete, specific answer when, in fact, the answer is "it depends on a number of factors." There is no one, correct, simple answer, in terms of hours, for adults. It is like asking *"How tall are men?"* and getting the answer 5 foot 7 inches (maybe close to average world-wide) and being satisfied with that value. Perhaps, more at issue is the question of *"How tall should men be?"* and get an answer of *at least 5 foot, 7 inches* making all shorter men feel that their height is a problematic issue when in fact, with respect to health, it is not (and maybe even be an advantage).

The CDC, the leading public health institute in the USA, seems to conclude that anything less than 7 hours of sleep per night is problematic, i.e., less than 7 hours of sleep is a public health issue. We imagine those of the CDC advocate 7 or more hours of sleep because they are aware that many adults are navigating their awake-time feeling tired and sleepy. This, in turn, leads to auto accidents (clearly a concern for an agency such as the CDC), falls and a contributor to many diseases. We imagine that those working at CDC presume their advice provides a nice, safe limit ensuring nearly all get adequate sleep. They do that, however, without considering that many persons who regularly sleep 6 hours and 30 minutes during 24 hours are often getting along just fine and faring as well as those getting 7 hours and 30 minutes of sleep-time.

This quest for a definitive answer to the question of *how many hours of sleep are necessary for being healthy* has put a portion of the population who are getting along just fine on 6 or so hours of sleep into a state of worry, when, in fact, they should not be worried or anxious. Also, those of advanced ages seem to need less sleep than others; however, they may worry if they are getting less than 7 hours of sleep a night, and perhaps, needlessly.

A more sensible, practical way of judging if you are getting adequate sleep is a personal answer rather than one based on national averages. If you awaken without an event wakening you (such as an alarm), feeling rested and refreshed, it is likely that you are getting adequate sleep *for you*. This is particularly the case if that is done regularly.

Please know that people getting an adequate amount of sleep do not just bounce out of bed and break into song and dance, they take a little time while awakening to gain full consciousness and stretch a bit before feeling alert. In brief, if you awaken after about 6 hours of sleep and feel eventually like dancing, you are just fine, maybe better than just fine.

However, if you feel like dancing after your usual 6 hours of sleeping and are a careful person, you may worry about not getting 7 or more hours of sleep. That worry may be because you have learned that less than 7 hours of sleep is problematic (from experts who mimic the CDC's advice). That worry and anxiety can set into motion a disturbance of what was healthy sleep into something more problematic. Worry and anxiety disturb sleep.

If you were getting restful sleep on less than 7 hours of sleep-time during a full day, don't worry. It is wise to conclude that you had enough sleep. It would be a disaster: If you were getting along just fine on 6 hours of sleep and you felt compelled to sleep 7 or more hours due to faulty recommendations. If you then decided to take sleeping pills to treat your *supposed* lack of sleep, you would cause yourself to have further health problems. This would especially be the case if you decided to take sleeping pills which suppress REM-sleep, are addictive and cause daytime sleepiness as well as other issues (see the sections on sleeping pills). After reading the first part of this book, you know: The regular use of sleeping pills can eventually lead to a host of problems.

Participants' Questions

If we were in a person to person consultation, it is imagined that a participant might ask about related topics to the question of how much sleep is necessary. A participant might ask, for example: "Is it O.K. to not get your daily quota of sleep all at one time? I get sleepy in mid-afternoon and I like to take a nap then. I awaken from my nap feeling refreshed."

The consultant's answer might be something like this: "If you have the luxury of being able to take a nap in the afternoon and you feel refreshed after your nightly sleep and after your nap, I see no reason for you to change your schedule. It is, indeed, a luxury to be able to sleep whenever you feel sleepy and tired. If, however, you need to be alert throughout the afternoon, being tired in the afternoon indicates you might lengthen you sleep-time during your regular time for sleep."

Napping can complement your previous night of sound sleep which may be why some cultures encourage siestas after lunch. A nap should be short. It is not meant to make up for an entire sleep deficit.[42] In fact, long naps may interfere with the ordinary circadian rhythm.

Once again, the standard for a "good night's sleep" is whether your feel refreshed and rested. Typically, if you are sleepy when you should not be, then a change in your sleep-schedule is in order. We will have more to say about this when we work with you as we set up an optimal sleep-schedule.

Chronic Insomnia

A counselor might take this opportunity to point out that there is a meaningful difference between acute insomnia and chronic insomnia. The cure for acute insomnia is merely to have the opportunity to sleep subsequent to a period of missing some sleep. It is natural to have a sleep debt and when that happens, you feel a need to sleep and when given the opportunity to sleep, you likely will sleep.

Chronic insomnia involves something more serious and it involves not getting restful, restorative sleep regularly. Chronic insomnia is a risk for multiple diseases including Alzheimer's disease.

Chronic insomnia usually develops over time and is characterized by frequent days of disturbed sleep. It is characterized by often being tired and irritable during the afternoon. Often there is a desire for healthy sleep, but circumstances seem to interfere. Among the common circumstances that are interfering with sound sleep is worry, anxiety, and rumination that seems to be almost habit-like, almost obsessive. The disturbances produced by these negative thoughts prevent healthy sleep, which, in turn reduce cognitive skills. Because the chronic insomnia does not seem to go away, the sufferer may come to the conclusion that they have *a disease* and seek a medicine to regularly get "a good night's sleep." If you have been following the contents of this book, you should be aware that this decision might not be a good choice and often may lead to less healthy sleep (e.g., a poor balance between REM and nonREM sleep) and generally poorer overall health.

The cure for chronic insomnia is a process, an activity and it takes some time and effort. The alternative is to hope that a sleeping pill will do the work of curing your chronic insomnia, clearly a false hope. A sleeping pill may induce a loss of consciousness that seems like natural sleep, but that kind of drug does not induce restorative sleep.

If you suffer from chronic insomnia, there are activities that you can engage during your awake-time that will be helpful at your time to sleep. One of those activities is to attend to the physical space in which you usually sleep, usually a bedroom. Another of those activities is to practice relaxing on cue. Relaxing on cue involves practicing a routine that will allow you to command yourself to relax when you wish to relax rather than being anxious or stressed. We shall advise you on a method that has been known to establish the ability to relax when you may need to relax rather than be troubled by emergent, unhelpful anxiety or fear.

Arrange Your Bedroom for Sleep

It is important that where you sleep is conducive to optimal sleep. We anticipate that there are a number of attributes of your bedroom that may have, over the years, become less than optimal. The following questions address these issues.

Questions

For each question, please pick the one answer that *best describes your situation.*

2. Do you have a TV in your bedroom?
                                a. Yes   b. No

3. Do you use modern electronics, e.g., a smartphone in the bedroom?   a. Yes   b. No

4. Can you darken your bedroom?
                                a. No   b. Yes

5. Can you arrange to make your bedroom cool in the evening?   a. No   b. Yes

6. Does the room have access to clean air and little noise?   a. No   b. Yes

7. Are your bed and bedsheets comfortable?

a. No   b. Yes

Answers

If you answered the questions in this section with **a**, you are not creating an ideal place to sleep.

Consultation

Your bedroom should be a sanctuary. The place where you sleep needs to be a place of calm, peace, privacy, and comfort.

Take some time to imagine what would make your bedroom a sanctuary for you. Each person differs in what they find to be comfortable. What color walls do you like? What sounds are pleasing and relaxing to you, if any? What kind of décor do you have? Take steps toward making your bedroom an ideal place for sleep and sensuality.

If you have sufficient financial resources, it makes good sense to arrange for a room to be used exclusively for sleep and sex. If you don't have spare cash, try to arrange a place so that there's a clear visual and mental separation between where you work and resolve problems and where you sleep.

The very act of improving your bedroom is conducive to getting a good night's sleep. It is satisfying to improve one's sleeping arrangements, even if it can only be done one small step at a time.

Simply making changes to your bedroom may alleviate some cases of insomnia and will also help sustain healthy sleep once you have recovered from any insomnia.

Lighting

Regardless of the hours your obligations allow you to sleep, your bedroom needs to be dark when you are ready for sleep, mimicking nighttime. If it cannot be darkened by shielding the room from light, then comfortable blindfolds can be used. Also, it is nice upon awakening to open the blinds and let in natural light.

During the time before for lying down to sleep, dim lighting entrains the action of melatonin, a neurotransmitter that ordinarily becomes more abundant when nighttime approaches. There is research to suggest making the lighting in your bedroom red just before going to bed.

Avoid Using Electronics Before Bedtime.

By their very nature, entertainment and advertisements are designed to arouse and focus your attention. Consequently, having a TV in your bedroom can present the opposite of developing a calm sanctuary for sleep and intimacy. The place where you sleep is not a place to check your e-mails or handle stressful phone conversations. Fortunately, the activities allowed by these electronic devices can easily be postponed. Your e-mails will still be available when you are outside of the bedroom and modern technology allows you to record any TV program you wish to view. Your telephone can take a message which you can listen to when you are awake. The morning news is nearly the same as the nightly news.

In a controlled study, healthy adults were tested to see the effect on sleep of reading a book on an iPad vs reading a print version.[43] Compared to those reading the book in print, they found that those reading the book on the iPad had suppressed melatonin release by over 50 percent and thus took longer to fall asleep. Sleep quality was also affected in addition to their sleep quantity. They spent a shorter time in REM sleep and felt tired and sleepy throughout the day following use of the iPad. Furthermore, there was a continuous delay in melatonin release for several days after extensive use of the iPad had stopped.

It is advised that you not use any electronic devices at least 2 hours before bedtime so as to not suppress melatonin release which signals that it is time to sleep. If you must use electronic devices just before sleep, consider installing software on your devices to gradually dim the arousing blue LED light emitted by your screen.

Temperature

Keep the temperature of the room relatively cool; around 65°F as this has been shown in sleep studies to promote higher quality sleep.[44] Comfort is controlled by bed clothes and blankets.

Clean Air

If the air inside your bedroom is foul, you can buy an air filter to cleanse the air in your bedroom, removing toxins and unwanted odors. House plants are also helpful in keeping the air clean.

Comfortable Bedding

Be sure to arrange for a comfortable bed, nice bed sheets and good pillows.

The Skill to Relax on Cue

We wish you to start the practice that will eventually be helpful in curing your chronic insomnia. We wish you to learn the skill by practicing the skill during your awake-time so that the developed skill can be deployed during the time when you are preparing to sleep. The rationale underlying the process is rather straightforward. Being relaxed is just the opposite of being tense, super-alert, anxious, fearful and unnecessarily angry. Being relaxed is helpful to the process of just drifting off to sleep. Evoking relaxation when maladaptive anxieties and fears are seemingly automatically emerging actually counters the maladaptive emotionality that may be a characteristic of chronic insomnia. In brief, being able to relax when you think that is useful, but may be difficult to do, is a very useful skill to have. Like most valuable skills it takes practice to learn the skill, but having learned the skill, it is very useful.

Technique to Relax on Cue

A technique used in CBTs-I is training for relaxation upon a self-designated cue. It was modeled after techniques developed by physiologists to help athletes relax rather than choke under pressure.

Wolpe adapted the technique to use in a therapy for maladaptive anxiety-fear.[45] The therapy was named systematic desensitization. Cued relaxation was used to counter-condition emergent anxiety-fear. Systematic desensitization is well-established as the preferred therapy for anxiety disorders, particularly for phobias.

This technique involves tensing and relaxing muscle groups throughout your body. Each time one relaxes a muscle-group, they should say the word "relax" in a calm tone of voice. When practicing this activity, the word "relax" will come to be the stimulus for an overall state of relaxation. The goal of the tense-relax practice is to be able to fully relax simply upon taking three deep breaths, slowly exhaling each breath and saying the word "relax" to oneself during the last slow, exhaled breath.

To be able to relax when needed is a useful technique in many situations; for example, prior to potential anxiety associated with a job interview or before addressing a large crowd.

With respect to treatment of insomnia, cued relaxation can be used to quell anxiety about not being able to go to sleep. Cued relaxation, like many skills, takes some time and practice to develop.

The following are instructions on how to develop the ability to relax on cue, that is, on your cue (i.e., when you take three deep breaths and say to yourself, relax). In this way, you can "turn on" relaxation prior to bedtime or at other moments you need to relax. The technique is relatively simple but must be practiced twice a day for at least two consecutive weeks to develop the ability to use the relaxation technique when needed. However, some are able to learn to relax on cue quicker.

First, commit yourself to the cue, i.e., take three deep breaths, then say the word "relax" in a calm manner. It is important that you associate the cue, with relaxation. History tells us that taking deep breaths is a way of controlling impulses and countering anxiety. Having determined a standard stimulus to condition to relaxation, we can begin a practice that will establish the action of relaxation upon using the cue.

Here's what you should do: Find a comfortable chair in a place where you won't be distracted. The first thing you should do is put your right arm straight out in front of you and tightly make a fist. Hold that tightened fist until it feels slightly uncomfortable (about 5 seconds) then say "relax" and release the tension. Take a moment to focus on how the relaxed muscles feel. Then, do the same thing with your left arm.

Flex your right bicep. Hold that contracted bicep for ten seconds or so. Then say "relax" and release the tension of that bicep. Feel the difference between the relaxed state and tensed state. Repeat with your left bicep.

Next, crunch your shoulders by moving your right shoulder toward your ear. Hold that contraction for about 10 seconds. Then say "relax" and release the tension in your shoulder. Once again, feel the difference. You may repeat this a couple times before doing the left shoulder the same way.

The next thing you should do is crunch your toes on your right foot like you were clenching your fist for a few seconds. Then say "relax" and release the tension in your toes. Feel the relaxation there as well. Then do the same on the left foot.

Next you should tense the calf of your right leg. Hold it for 10 seconds or so. Then you should relax it. Feel the relaxation, then do your left calf muscle the same way.

Contract your right quad (muscle in the top of your thigh). Once again hold that for a few seconds, then relax. Feel the relaxation, then do the same with your left quad.

Next contract your right glutes (buttocks). Continue to hold the tension for a few seconds and say the word "relax" upon relaxing the muscle. Repeat this exercise with your left glutes.

Then tense to the abdominal muscles. Hold the tension in your stomach muscles for about 10 seconds. Say the word "relax" upon relaxing the abdominal muscles.

Continue to follow the pattern with the muscles in your chest, then relax. Then, make a funny face by contracting the muscles in your forehead tightly and puckering your lips. Then relax the tightened face. Do that a few times. Each time, focusing on the feeling of relaxation that comes after you say "relax."

Next, tighten the muscles in the back of your neck (point your chin toward the sky) hold that for 10 seconds and then relax. Remember to say "relax" each time you relax a muscle group.

At this point you've completed your first round of cued-relaxation. You will need to do this often before you have fully learned what it feels like to be relaxed and can engage this practice on cue. However, once learned the ability to relax on your conscious command, it is a valuable tool to have.

You can test yourself to see if you've learned how to relax on cue. We recommend you use the cue of taking three deeps breaths and then say the word "relax". Sit in a chair and think of something that makes you anxious. Once you have that in mind, take three deep breaths and say relax. If you sense some diminution in your perceived anxiety, you're making progress in your counter-conditioning of perceived anxiety. If you don't see a difference, practice makes perfect, continue to practice.

We recommend that you do this practice for cued relaxation at different times of the day and in different places. In other words, not in the same place so that you only learn to relax there, but not everywhere. Once you can successfully quell an imagined anxiety, the next thing to do is try it at bedtime.

Sleep and Anxiety

There are two kinds of anxiety that may interfere with getting a good night's sleep. There is what is called *generalized anxiety*. Generalized anxiety is worrying, fretting and ruminating about all kinds of potential unpleasantries and is not specific to one circumstance. We have some comments on generalized anxiety later in the book.

Here, we address the anxiety that emerges as one lies awake without seemingly being able to go to sleep. For want of a better term, we are going to call this kind of anxiety a bed-bedroom phobia.

Bed-bedroom Phobias

Here are some comments that an individual might make who becomes anxious as bedtime approaches.

I dread lying awake, night after night.

I feel awful, because I don't sleep well.

I'm not going to be ready for tomorrow.

If I don't sleep, I will get sick.

This lack of sleep will affect my obligations.

Questions

9. Are the statements given above similar to the ones you might make?
    a. Yes, I say similar things when I talk to myself.
    b. Yes, occasionally I say things like that but not characteristically.
    c. No.

10. When preparing for bedtime, I have the following thoughts and feelings.
    a. I become anxious about facing another night of poor sleep and worry about how it will affect the next day.

b. I sometimes worry about how long it takes me to fall asleep.
c. I usually do not have many thoughts about my sleeping, I just go to bed and then I fall asleep.

Answers

Those answering **a** are expressing a serious concern. Those answering **a**, even if your thoughts are only similar, will likely profit from reading on. Those answering **b** may also learn some interesting information that might be useful in preventing a bed-bedtime phobia.

Consultation

What is a phobia? A phobia is the development of fear and/or anxiety associated with a specific place or thing (a common phobia is fear of spiders).

It may seem strange that a person might develop a phobia to one's own bed, the preparation for sleep or merely lying down to sleep. Actually, it is not so strange. The process of developing a phobia is a very adaptive process that is well-developed among us all. When an anxiety or fearful emotional wells up (a response) in the presence of a recognizable event (a stimulus), the pairing of the fear-like emotion tends to *automatically* become associated with the situation. It is built into us, the perception of danger (manifest as anxiety or fear) from any situation should incite moving away from danger. In other words, we seek safety readily in face of anxiety and fear provided there is a safe place to go. And, if there is any real pain or cognitive pain is experienced in the situation, the association with the negative experience and situation becomes very strong, very quickly.

Obviously, it is very adaptive to avoid situations that evoke anxiety, fear and especially pain and to have the avoidance response readily available when the situation again comes into play.

As one prepares for and eventually lies down to sleep, a number of conditions, including anxiety producing thoughts might emerge. Also, sometimes pain including physical pain due to disease or injury and thoughts of social pain can emerge when lying down. Even something as innocuous as drinking too many caffeinated beverages before trying to sleep can evoke an alertness and anxiety that is the opposite of being calm and drifting off to sleep. When anxiety is experienced consistently at bedtime, an association between the anxiety and the bedroom is formed. That is, when the pairings of stimulus: bed; and response: anxiety occur together, a conditional anxiety can be established. Further that conditioned response can be very enduring. When these conditions prevail, you have inadvertently, established a phobia, a fear elicited by being in bed and not getting to sleep. Further, the phobia itself hinders going to sleep. *The result is a nightly battle between the strength and duration of the anxiety and the physiological need to sleep, a stressful situation that tends to be self-perpetuating and manifested as chronic insomnia.*

Once this association (to bed and anxiety) is established, the bond between trying to sleep and anxiety about getting to sleep becomes stronger. When such associations become engrained, whether they are adaptive or not, they tend to become so automatic that they are elicited unconsciously. That presents a problem. It becomes difficult to call up how and why the habit was established. Further, it is difficult to talk yourself out of any habit, but particularly out of any habit involving anxiety and fear. When the conditioning is well-established and when the stimulus for anxiety appears, the response is automatic and not under the person's rational control. Telling yourself, "I am not going to be anxious about getting to sleep tonight" and expect your thinking to resolve your insomnia will merely be a disappointing source of more anxiety.

Given the intractability of your phobia, you might even resign yourself to the possibility that you have a disease deserving a strong medicine. Given that possibility, the temptation to take a sleeping pill can be strong. A sleeping pill might induce unconsciousness rather quickly when in bed. If that happens, you will also have the automatic association of taking a pill and getting some sense of relief. The relief strengthens pill-taking. As mentioned, the usual hypnotics are at best a brief solution to an enduring problem eventually made worse by the drugs interfering with the normal cycle of sleep. Further, the actions of the pill do not overcome the phobia that has been established. That is, when you stop taking the pill, your phobia will rebound with the associated anxiety.

In brief, phobic-like anxiety about not being able to get to sleep or sustain sleep is not a logical problem, it is a *psychological* problem. The resolution lies in psychological procedures that have been shown to be effective and are embodied in modern cognitive behavioral therapy.

Managing a Bed-Bedroom Phobia

There are, at least, two ways of managing a bed-bedroom phobia. A way is to replace the emergent anxiety with a response opposite of anxiety (called counter-conditioning). Another way is to change the situation so that the usual stimuli that evokes the anxiety are no longer present. We will discuss each approach. They are not mutually exclusive and can be used together or separately.

Counter-Conditioning

In a previous section, we advised you to do exercises to develop the skill to relax on cue. Using that skill, you can counter the anxiety that sustains a bed-bedroom phobia.

There are other activities you should do. We advise you to think about your usual steps you take as you are preparing for bed, getting into bed, assuming a comfortable position in bed, and then taking some time to drift off to sleep.

We will advise you now and later when we discuss the optimal schedule of preparing for sleep and sleeping that you engage the same routine every time you are preparing to get into bed.

Note: the usual time that it takes for most people from the time they get into bed to when they are asleep is about 15 minutes. You might think of segments of these 15 minutes as an early time, a middle time and the beginning of sleep time.

The procedure is straightforward. The first thing you might do is take off your usual clothes in preparation for going to bed. If that is the case, designate that as step one in a progression of steps toward the start of sleeping.

As you begin preparing for bed and have a sense of emergent anxiety, you immediately evoke your learned cue to relax. That is, when a dread of getting into bed is experienced, you do your cue: you take three deep breaths and slowly exhale with each breath and then say relax using the same tone as when practicing the skill of relaxing on cue. If after you evoke the learned cue to relax and you again feel dread of going to bed emerge, repeat the learned skill of relaxing again: deep breathing followed by the word relax and actually becoming relaxed. You do this with the early part of your routine of getting ready for bed until during that early activity you feel relaxed rather than anxious.

Then, engage the next step toward getting ready for bed and you may again feel anxious. Again, use your practiced skill by breathing slowly and saying the word relax. You repeat the counter-conditioning with each step until you are actually relaxed and do not feel anxiety. Note: your initial steps toward going to sleep (first steps toward preparing to go to bed) are usually not the most intense experiences of anxiety about not getting enough sleep. Nevertheless, given your personal history, it may be necessary to take some time and effort to relax as you approach the time to go to bed. Please take the time. Become relaxed before the separate steps for getting into bed.

There are things most people do before retiring to bed. They include activities such as urinating, brushing your teeth, arranging the bed. Others bathe or shower before bedtime. You probably have a set of activities you often use. The basic idea is to relax with each step toward climbing in bed, particularly if you feel any emerging anxiety.

It is a tradition in some cultures to pray before retiring and we often teach our children to affirm their gratitude for parents and those who look after them. Now, we are not sure that such activity is helpful in overcoming chronic insomnia. However, in addition to countering any emergent anxiety by evoking your learned skill at relaxing, you might say this widely used affirmation. Just before climbing in bed, say to yourself or out-loud "Grant me the serenity to accept the things I cannot change, the courage to change the things I can and the wisdom to know the difference."

A Daytime way to Reduce Sleep Anxiety

Now if the procedure described above appears to be a bit cumbersome or disruptive, there is an alternative. It can be done any time during the day when you have a few moments by yourself in a comfortable chair. Once in the chair, close your eyes, and imagine the first step toward getting into bed. When you imagine the first step and feel some anxiety, counter that anxiety with your skill at relaxing. When you imagine that first step again and feel emerging anxiety, again, relax. When you have countered the anxiety with the first step, then, in your imagination, take the imagined next step toward going to sleep. Counter-condition any anxiety that may emerge by relaxing all of your muscles as you have learned to do when you evoke your cue. Let your imagination continue, step by step, until you imagine being in bed and free of troublesome anxiety.

You might conclude that doing the counter-conditioning merely using your imagination and your learned skill at relaxing on cue will not transfer to the time when you are actually going to bed and not getting to sleep. Interestingly, the research indicates that imaging anxiety and counter-conditioning that imagined anxiety is remarkably effective and is helpful in reducing phobias.

Your Time Just Before Sleeping

While you may have climbed into bed in a relaxed state, there might be a resurgence of anxiety about not falling asleep quickly. Unfortunately, those negative thoughts induce more anxiety. That alertness-anxiety is the opposite of just quietly, calmly drifting off to sleep. When that happens, you can counter the emerging anxiety with your skill of relaxing on cue.

This is a good place to note, again, that, on average, healthy sleepers (those not having chronic insomnia and probably you before you developed chronic insomnia) take about 15 minutes to drift off to sound sleep. A relaxed state upon getting into bed may not be sufficient. There might be an emergence of anxiety rather than being patient and letting your natural need for sleep progress. When in bed and again feeling anxious and having unsettling thoughts, you may evoke relaxation. You evoke relaxation while at same time just gently moving your thoughts to as much as nothing as you can; just no specific thoughts as much as you can arrange, a sort of calm, not thinking about much of anything. It can be helpful to turn your attention solely to your breathing. Now, this is a difficult state to maintain. When your thoughts again drift toward worrisome things, notice the troubling thought, and then just gently again move your thinking toward no thoughts. Notice only your breathing as again you relax as you have learned to do. You let sleep take over. Fortunately, your inherent need to sleep will help you go to sleep.

Fearing Loss of Consciousness

Sleep involves losing consciousness; something that happens to every person almost every 24-hour period, i.e., you drift off to sleep. Sleep does not mean that you are totally unaware of real dangers (e.g., smoke from fire; smoke & fire alarms; strange, loud noises; babies crying; poor breathing, etc.). Real dangers ordinarily awaken sleepers. It is only when drugged by sleeping pills, excessive alcohol-intake, opioid pain-killers in excess, and such that individuals totally lose consciousness and cannot awaken when the need arises. These drugs produce something akin to a coma, not something akin to sleep. A far too common event is a drunken person decides to smoke a cigarette before going to sleep and is so tired and sleepy that the person falls asleep with a lit cigarette and that sets the bed on fire. The drunk may be so wiped out that even a bed on fire is not sufficient to waken the person until the situation is beyond correcting.

Our biology demands that we sleep, but that same biology does not make us totally unaware when asleep. We evolved in a world of predators and we survived as a species by being aroused by real dangers. Modern humans are by virtue of being descendants of a long-line of prepared sleepers usually awaken to danger. Modern people have the same ability as our ancestors, except when drugged.

A restoration of healthy sleep actually allows for prepared sleep, i.e., sleep that *is not* akin to coma but *is sleep* that is protective and restorative. Healthy sleep allows for REM and nonREM sleep and a sufficient amount of sleep allowing you to awaken feeling refreshed and ready for activity that will sustain you, i.e., eating, drinking, providing for your needs, being an active member of your social group, etc.

In brief, among the safest things you can do daily is to drift off to sleep, i.e., lose an awareness of self but not lose some basic alertness that is characteristic of "a good night's sleep." In turn, that healthy sleep provides the means, upon awakening, to think more clearly, to adapt to new challenges, and to sustain those habits that have served you well and to change those habits that are maladaptive.

If you have read the above, you have the information to overcome your insomnia. Merely knowing that information is not sufficient. You have to engage the activities to permanently cure your insomnia by developing a habit of daily healthy sleep. It is something you have to do yourself. No known medicine can magically induce healthy sleep. No one can talk you into sleeping well if you have chronic insomnia. Merely being told you have insomnia does not help, you probably already are well aware of that. Social support is helpful, but only in the sense that it encourages you to do the activities you need to do to cure your chronic insomnia.

If you are a partner of a person suffering from insomnia that is working toward curing their insomnia, please be tolerant of the rather time-consuming work that will eventually allow efficiency in getting to sleep. If you are the sufferer of chronic insomnia, you can explain that I must do something about my insomnia and please support me in my activities to develop new habits supporting healthy sleep. Your chronic insomnia most likely was a bit troublesome to you partner and seeing you work toward a resolution to the problem will be a good thing for both of you.

Change the Stimuli Associated with Insomnia

Recall that at the beginning of our discussion of how to counter the anxiety that is interfering with sleep, we mentioned that there was another way of reducing the anxiety that had developed, and, in turned sustained insomnia. Here is a brief discussion of this second way.

The stimuli (the circumstances) of bed and bedroom phobia is the bed and bedroom. You can remodel your sleeping place so that it is clearly different than the one in which you developed your phobia, hence reducing the stimuli that induced and sustained the anxiety about a loss of a "good night's sleep."

Note among the things we asked you to do is to make your sleeping space a sanctuary. Those changes may involve reducing some of the relevant stimuli evoking anxiety about not getting to sleep in a reasonable time. That involves doing things such as removing the TV, getting new bedding, and other activities that are likely to be interfering with good sleep.

If nothing else seems to work at reducing anxiety about getting to sleep in an orderly fashion, then you might take the action of completely remodeling the bedroom. Paint the walls, change the lighting, get new bedding, get new sleep clothes, etc. If you have the opportunity, go to a different bedroom in your home and see if going to bed there is helpful. If you have little or no trouble getting to sleep in a hotel room when traveling, then you know that it is time to change the features of your bedroom.

Establish a Schedule for Optimal Sleep

It is a consensus of those who do research on sleeping and those who write books,[3,42,45-47] on the topic that it is extraordinarily helpful to establish a habitual routine when preparing to sleep and when to going sleep. We will provide advice on a very good way to arrange a schedule for optimal sleep.

The consensus advice is to rigorously sustain a schedule for optimal sleep for as much as 6 weeks in order to completely overcome chronic insomnia. Taking the time and effort to overcome your insomnia will provide you the overall skills to manage insomnia and that is a good investment. It pays off in the long-run, because, once you have the skills to deal with insomnia, you probably will never again experience insomnia due to cognitive, behavioral issues. You will know how to manage any return of insomnia and do so with ease.

The optimal schedule for sleep will help you to do the activities that will be helpful in overcoming insomnia. The schedule is like a developed plan to cure your chronic insomnia or prevent insomnia if you have yet to be troubled by not getting a "good night's sleep."

Questions

11. Do you need an alarm to wake up nearly every morning?

a. Yes, I usually awaken to an alarm and it always seems to be mildly irritating.

b. I sometimes need an alarm when the circumstance requires me to awaken before I usually do.

c. No, I usually awaken without an alarm or get up before my alarm goes off.

12. Do you sleep-in during the weekend?

a. Yes, I need that time to refresh and catch up on my sleep and I do sleep-in on weekends. I try to repay my hours of lost sleep (my sleep-debt) during the weekend by spending more time in bed and sleeping. If circumstances prevent that time (extra opportunity to sleep) during the weekend, I am irritated.

b. Yes, sometimes, particularly when I have pleasant social occasions scheduled for Friday or Saturday nights.

c. No, I awaken at my usual time and I like that because I enjoy my weekends.

13. Do you fall asleep or yawn excessively during boring activities (e.g., dull lectures, uninspiring meetings, during TV commercials, etc.)?

a. Yes, I struggle with this often.

b. Sometimes, I nod off during boring events and if it is an important event, it is embarrassing when I nod off.

c. No, I usually just power through the boring parts of the day, often faking an interest which sometimes overcomes the boredom.

Answers

If you are answering these three questions with a positive answer (the **c** choice), then you are probably already doing things well and should continue with your daily routines. However, if you answer the questions with **a**, that indicates a problematic situation. Read the following consultation for ways of correcting the problem.

If you answer the questions with **b**, you may benefit from reading the following consultation.

Consultation

There is a strong possibility that you have not arranged your world in a way that allows for a period of healthy sleep, especially during the work-week. Here, the focus is on rearranging your schedule. We are going to advise what may seem strange at first, but this schedule has considerable advantages.

To execute CBTs-I well, one must arrange for a detailed schedule for sleeping that is practiced for as long as six weeks.

Here is an example of someone's schedule. Jess is a banker and has a regular schedule that requires her to be at work every weekday at 8 am. Her commute to work is at most 30 minutes, so she usually makes sure she leaves her home at 7.30 am. Upon awakening, she allows herself an hour each day for toileting, cleaning herself, getting dressed, preparing and eating breakfast. She has this routine well-established and it runs efficiently. This would mean setting her alarm to wake her up at 6:30 am; her first reminder of the day. We prefer the word "reminder" rather than "alarm," for starting a morning routine is nothing to be alarmed about. It is the signal to prepare to leave her home in an hour.

Jess can return to her home some 9.5 to 10 hours after she left it (30 min to work, 4 hours of work, 30 min for lunch, 4 more hours of work—

since Jess is a conscientious worker, she often works another 30 min–and 30 min to return home). To implement a schedule designed to establish healthy sleep and to correct chronic insomnia, the advice is to establish a new schedule of when to go to bed.

To give herself 8 hours of opportunity to sleep, she needs to be in bed 8 hours before she must awaken, i.e., in Jess's case 10:30 pm. For some, their nightly routine, i.e., preparing to go to bed, may span 15 min-30 min depending on a person's preferences. To stop activities of your ordinary awake time, we recommend that you have a reminder. We realize that this is unusual; Having an alarm to go to bed as well as an alarm to awaken. If all goes well, that "alarm" will turn into a gentle reminder to start your pre-bedtime routine.

In order to prepare for bed, it is recommended that there be a fixed routine that is done in a fixed order. Recall that we encouraged a fixed routine when detailing how to counter-condition any anxiety you experience as you prepare to go into bed.

Some may use this time to turn on environmental cues for relaxation such as certain quiet music, calming scents (e.g., lavender mist), and avoid bright lighting.

Having a fixed routine, the skill to relax on cue, having prepared your living space for optimal sleep, and then attending to all of this for 6 weeks will, most likely, resolve chronic insomnia.

The Value of this Routine

Recall, we discussed the issue of how much sleep is necessary. The conclusion was it depends on whether you awaken feeling restored and ready for a day of activities. We imagine that many of you, once you manage your insomnia, will awaken before the 8 hours allocated for sleep and before the reminder to arouse from sleep. This time between the end of sleep and the start of getting ready for the day's activities is a bonus. It is a good time to engage the extra effort to prepare for a particularly delicious breakfast, do some stretching exercises, or watch your favorite late-night TV program that you recorded. This alert time is also a good time to do planning and rational problem solving; a much-improved approach over trying to solve problems when sleepy and tired.

It helps to keep a record of your activities during your six-week program of sleep-improvement. A guide for keeping a record is in the appendix. You can add to it by keeping a more comprehensive diary. A diary has a utility of having you notice signs of progress.

Other Issues that Might Need Attention

We have yet to discuss with you some other issues that may be associated with your sleep.

Waking Up in the Middle of a Sleep-Period

Waking up once in the middle of a sleep-period (usually during the night) is not something that should interfere with having healthy sleep. This is particularly the case if you have allocated a full eight hours of time to get "a good night's sleep." Individuals often awaken in the middle of the night to urinate. Needing to urinate frequently a symptom of problems such as type 2 diabetes. As a consequence of the necessity to not wet the bed, you should develop the construal to not fret about the necessity to wake up, but to have the mindset that is conducive to getting back to sleep. You can use the same techniques that you might have employed when getting to sleep in the first place.

Going to the toilet in the middle of a sleep-period involves a remarkable increase in the likelihood of falling and breaking a bone especially if you're older. Moving in darkness when groggy can be dangerous. It is clearly prudent to make the pathway from the bed to the toilet as safe as possible. For example: remove throw rugs, store shoes and other objects that can cause one to stumble, i.e., move anything that might trip you out of the pathway. If there are stairs and doors between your bedroom and the toilet, attend to making that part of your path safe (e.g., have adequate lighting, not blindingly bright lighting, of course).

The experience of waking up many times during the night may be a symptom of sleep apnea. This symptom should be brought to the attention of medical personnel.

Exercise and Unusual Exercises

There is consensus: An activity one should do during the awake-period of the day (usually the daytime) is to engage a period of physical exercise that increases your breathing and your heart-rate. A regular routine of exercise of about 150 minutes during a week is clearly a health-promoting and health-sustaining activity. It is not surprising that such promotes better sleep. However, that period of exercise should not be just before you get into bed. Before getting into bed, as emphasized earlier, should be a time of calmly preparing to sleep.

There are specific exercises that one can do to manage snoring. There are descriptions of these exercises on the internet and there is no need to repeat them here.

There are specific exercises that one can engage to control the urge to urinate (preventing urinary incontinence). Again, there are descriptions of these exercises on the internet and no need to repeat them here. These exercises are named after the individual that popularized such, hence called Kegel exercises

While the information is freely available on the internet, please be aware that these sites often have strong ties to commercial activity, including the commercial activity of providing medical care.

Anxiety and Depression

Insomnia is often accompanied by generalized anxiety disorder or major depression or both anxiety and depression. The question is which comes first, the insomnia or the other disorders? The answer is not known, probably because for some insomnia precedes the anxiety-depression and for others anxiety and depression induces insomnia. What is known is that successfully treating insomnia accompanied by anxiety-depression is helpful in managing the anxiety-depression.

Here is what we do know: the prescription of long-acting benzodiazepines is often not beneficial in treating generalized anxiety disorder, such can disrupt normal sleep, increase appetite that might lead to obesity and increases the risk of early death.[19,48] What we also know is that the prescription of the most commonly prescribed drugs for depression are of only marginally beneficial.[49] There are cognitive behavioral therapies shown to be effective in treating anxiety and depression.

This is not the place to discuss the details of how to treat anxiety and depression. But you should know that some of the skills you have learned while managing your insomnia can be deployed in dealing with anxiety and depression as well.

Cued relaxation was developed to counter-condition phobias and is remarkably effective with simple phobias. Recall, we suggested deploying it to manage bed-bedroom phobias associated with managing chronic insomnia. The ability to relax on cue is generally useful in calming stress and surely could be used in the service of reducing stressful thoughts.

The late extraordinarily skilled research scientist who focused on depression, particularly among women, Susan Nolen-Hoeksema, focused on the propensity of those depressed to ruminate and overthink previous and potential disturbing circumstances. This rumination and overthinking are often critical of the person doing the rumination and overthinking. This kind of thinking sustains depressive episodes and may even be an initiator of depression.

For more comprehensive information on controlling maladaptive thinking, we suggest any of the books written for the general public by Professor Nolen-Hoeksema.[50,51]

Thought-stopping

There is a broad general idea (a construal) that is useful to recall when ruminating. That is, *there is no way to change the past. The only thing you have control over is the future.* And, there is the new understanding, brain plasticity, that confirms that one has more control over the future than previously believed. That is, your behavior can change your brain in the service of developing healthy habits.

The thought-stopping technic is remarkably simple, but remarkably effective. When you become aware of rumination, overthinking, dwelling on unproductive thinking, here is what you do. Take the fingers of your hand and press them against your forehead. When done, then: In a commanding voice (either out loud or to yourself) yell, STOP! Then: swipe your hand from your forehead to a trash bin (it can be an imagined trash bin) throwing the unpleasant thought away from you. Then: immediately think a nice thought, can be any kind of nice thought, a favorite food, a favorite song, a pleasant reminder of a nice event.

If you address rumination in this way repeatedly you will find a diminution in thinking worthless thoughts.

Mindfulness

There is a well-known technic that has become increasingly popular as a way of limiting stress and generalized anxiety; mindfulness. Its popularity has been shown by recent research to be well-earned. Similar to other cognitive, behavioral procedures, mindfulness technics take some practice to achieve the calming effects that reduce stress and needless worry and anxiety. Because of mindfulness being popular, there are a host of books and websites that present the technics of mindfulness. They are adequate for learning enough about mindfulness to be helpful and often the lessons are freely given or given with modest payments (e.g., by inexpensive books). We suggest that if you are experiencing generalize anxiety, manifest as rumination and worry, that learning to practice mindfulness will be of benefit.

Summary

Sleep is vital. Efficient sleep, "a good night's sleep," is refreshing and restorative. Poor sleep hinders being healthy and happy.

Poor sleep, insomnia and related problems, got that way because they got that way. However, just because they got that way does not mean that you need to live the rest of your life that way. Insomnia and related problems can be overcome by doing activities that will develop efficient sleep. Healthy sleep can happen because it can get that way; because you can manage your mission toward habitual, healthy sleep. The good circumstance is that you can take charge of a vital part of your life and have that sleep-period of your 24-hour day to be in the service of your health and happiness.

Yes, the mission of restoring healthy sleep, once disrupted, may seem like a rather arduous, tedious journey. However, as you "travel" that mission, the steps will become easier and easier. You learn to recognize dangers and skillfully avoid them. You learn to question exaggerated claims given by those more interested in making money than in your long-term health and happiness.

You can prevail! Your natural tendency to sleep daily is your friend and, like a good friend, will help you to prevail.

References

1. Reid LD, Taylor DZ, Walf AA. *Cognitive behavioural therapy (CBT) use in Alzheimer's disease: mitigating risks associated with the olfactory brain.* In: V. Reedy (Ed.), *The Neuroscience of Dementia*, Book 2, Cambridge, MA, Elsevier, 2019. (in press).

2. Reid LD, Avens FE, Walf AA. Cognitive behavioral therapy (CBT) for preventing Alzheimer's disease. *Behav Brain Res.* 2017;334:163-177. doi:10.1016/j.bbr.2017.07.024

3. Walker M. *Why We Sleep Unlocking the Power of Sleep and Dreams.* New York, NY: Scribner; 2017.

4. Nedergaard M. Garbage truck of the brain. *Science.* 2013;340(6140):1529-1530. doi:10.1126/science.1240514

5. Chong YY, Fryar CD, Gu Q. *Prescription sleep aid use among adults: United States, 2005-2010.* Hyattsville, MD: National Center for Health Statistics; 2013. https://www.cdc.gov/nchs/products/databriefs/db127.htm. Accessed July 30, 2018.

6. Billioti de Gage S, Moride Y, Ducruet T, et al. Benzodiazepine use and risk of Alzheimer's disease: case-control study. *BMJ.* 2014;349(sep09 2):g5205-g5205. doi:10.1136/bmj.g5205

7. Brandt J, Leong C. Benzodiazepines and Z-Drugs: An updated review of major adverse outcomes reported on in epidemiologic research. *Drugs RD.* 2017;17(4):493-507. doi:10.1007/s40268-017-0207-7

8. Donnelly K, Bracchi R, Hewitt J, Routledge PA, Carter B. Benzodiazepines, Z-drugs and the risk of hip fracture: A systematic review and meta-analysis. *PLOS ONE.* 2017;12(4):e0174730. doi:10.1371/journal.pone.0174730

9. Sakurai T, Amemiya A, Ishii M, et al. Orexins and orexin receptors: a family of hypothalamic neuropeptides and G protein-coupled receptors that regulate feeding behavior. *Cell.* 1998;92(4):573-585.

10. de Lecea L, Kilduff TS, Peyron C, et al. The hypocretins: hypothalamus-specific peptides with neuroexcitatory activity. *Proc Natl Acad Sci USA.* 1998;95(1):322-327.

11. BELSOMRA® (suvorexant) C-IV Works Differently. https://www.belsomra.com/belsomraworksdifferently/?src=google&med=cpc&camp=Belsomra. Accessed September 3, 2018.

12. Sateia MJ, Buysse DJ, Krystal AD, Neubauer DN, Heald JL. Clinical Practice Guideline for the Pharmacologic Treatment of Chronic Insomnia in Adults: An American Academy of Sleep Medicine Clinical Practice Guideline. *J Clin Sleep Med.* 2017;13(02):307-349. doi:10.5664/jcsm.6470

13. Skip new insomnia drug Belsomra - *Consumer Reports*. https://www.consumerreports.org/cro/news/2015/07/skip-new-insomnia-drug-belsomra/index.htm. Accessed September 3, 2018.

14. Pagel JF, Pandi-Perumal SR, Monti JM. Treating insomnia with medications. *Sleep Sci Pract*. 2018;2(1). doi:10.1186/s41606-018-0025-z

15. Kantor ED, Rehm CD, Du M, White E, Giovannucci EL. Trends in Dietary Supplement Use Among US Adults From 1999-2012. *JAMA*. 2016;316(14):1464. doi:10.1001/jama.2016.14403

16. Alghamdi BS. The neuroprotective role of melatonin in neurological disorders. *J Neurosci Res*. 2018;96(7):1136-1149. doi:10.1002/jnr.24220

17. Kripke DF, Langer RD, Kline LE. Hypnotics' association with mortality or cancer: a matched cohort study. *BMJ Open*. 2012;2(1):e000850. doi:10.1136/bmjopen-2012-000850

18. Weich S, Pearce HL, Croft P, et al. Effect of anxiolytic and hypnotic drug prescriptions on mortality hazards: retrospective cohort study. *BMJ*. 2014;348:g1996.

19. Kripke DF. Hypnotic drug risks of mortality, infection, depression, and cancer: but lack of benefit. *F1000Research*. 2016;5:918. doi:10.12688/f1000research.8729.1

20. Joya FL, Kripke DF, Loving RT, Dawson A, Kline LE. Meta-analyses of hypnotics and infections: eszopiclone, ramelteon, zaleplon, and zolpidem. *J Clin Sleep Med JCSM Off Publ Am Acad Sleep Med*. 2009;5(4):377-383.

21. Kinch MS, Haynesworth A, Kinch SL, Hoyer D. An overview of FDA-approved new molecular entities: 1827-2013. *Drug Discov Today*. 2014;19(8):1033-1039. doi:10.1016/j.drudis.2014.03.018

22. Research Center for Drug Evaluation and Research. Drug Applications for Over-the-Counter (OTC) Drugs. U.S. Food & Drug Administration. https://www.fda.gov/drugs/developmentapprovalprocess/howdrugsaredevelopedandapproved/approvalapplications/over-the-counterdrugs/default.htm. Accessed July 30, 2018.

23. Centers for Disease Control and Prevention. Deaths and Mortality. https://www.cdc.gov/nchs/fastats/deaths.htm. Published March 5, 2018. Accessed August 9, 2018.

24. Statistics on OTC Use. Consumer Healthcare Products Association. https://www.chpa.org/marketstats.aspx. Accessed August 7, 2018.

25. US Department of Health and Human Services. Dietary Supplement Health and Education Act of 1994. https://ods.od.nih.gov/About/DSHEA_Wording.aspx. Accessed August 19, 2018.

26. Consumer Advisory: Kava-Containing dietary supplements may be associated with severe liver injury. US Food and Drug Administration. https://wayback.archiveit.org/7993/20170722144010/https://www.fda.gov/Food/RecallsOutbreaksEmergencies/SafetyAlertsAdvisories/ucm085482.htm. Accessed August 7, 2018.

27. Maher RL, Hanlon J, Hajjar ER. Clinical consequences of polypharmacy in elderly. *Expert Opin Drug Saf.* 2014;13(1):57-65. doi:10.1517/14740338.2013.827660

28. *Health, United States 2016: With Chartbook on Long-Term Trends in Health.* National Center for Health Statistics. Hyattsville, MD. 2017 May. Report No.: 2017-1232.

29. Research TM. Global Mattress Market to be worth US$43.43 Billion by 2024 - TMR. GlobeNewswire News Room. http://globenewswire.com/newsrelease/2018/04/19/1481706/0/en/Global-Mattress-Market-to-be-worth-US-43-43-Billion-by-2024-TMR.html. Published April 19, 2018. Accessed August 7, 2018.

30. Brody JE. Studies Show Little Benefit in Supplements. *The New York Times.* https://www.nytimes.com/2016/11/15/well/eat/studies-show-little-benefit-in-supplements.html. Published April 8, 2018. Accessed August 19, 2018.

31. Lipton E. Hatch a 'Natural Ally' of Supplements Industry. *The New York Times.* https://www.nytimes.com/2011/06/21/us/politics/21hatch.html. Published June 20, 2011. Accessed August 19, 2018.

32. Free Image on Pixabay - Field Of Poppies, Thriving Mohnfeld. /en/field-of-poppies-thriving-mohnfeld-3432640/. Accessed October 27, 2018.

33. Piller C. Hidden conflicts? Science. 2018 6;361(6397):16-20. doi:10.1126/science.361.6397.16.

34. Morin CM, Hauri PJ, Espie CA, Spielman AJ, Buysse DJ, Bootzin RR. Nonpharmacologic treatment of chronic insomnia. An American Academy of Sleep Medicine review. *Sleep.* 1999;22(8):1134-1156.

35. Chesson AL, Anderson WM, Littner M, et al. Practice parameters for the nonpharmacologic treatment of chronic insomnia. An American Academy of Sleep Medicine report. Standards of Practice Committee of the American Academy of Sleep Medicine. *Sleep.* 1999;22(8):1128-1133.

36. Riemann D, Perlis ML. The treatments of chronic insomnia: A review of benzodiazepine receptor agonists and psychological and behavioral therapies. *Sleep Med Rev.* 2009;13(3):205-214. doi:10.1016/j.smrv.2008.06.001

37. Mitchell MD, Gehrman P, Perlis M, Umscheid CA. Comparative effectiveness of cognitive behavioral therapy for insomnia: a systematic review. *BMC Fam Pract.* 2012;13(1). doi:10.1186/1471-2296-13-40

38. Brasure M, Fuchs E, MacDonald R, et al. Psychological and behavioral interventions for managing insomnia disorder: An evidence report for a clinical practice guideline by the American College of Physicians. *Ann Intern Med.* 2016;165(2):113. doi:10.7326/M15-1782

39. Qaseem A, Kansagara D, Forciea MA, Cooke M, Denberg TD. Clinical guidelines committee of the American College of Physicians. Management of chronic insomnia disorder in adults: A Clinical practice guideline from the American College of Physicians. *Ann Intern Med.* 2016;165(2):125. doi:10.7326/M15-2175

40. Koffel E, Bramoweth AD, Ulmer CS. Increasing access to and utilization of cognitive behavioral therapy for insomnia (CBT-I): a narrative review. *J Gen Intern Med.* 2018;33(6):955-962. doi:10.1007/s11606-018-4390-1

41. Seyffert M, Lagisetty P, Landgraf J, et al. Internet-Delivered Cognitive Behavioral Therapy to Treat Insomnia: A Systematic Review and Meta-Analysis. *PloS One.* 2016;11(2):e0149139. doi:10.1371/journal.pone.0149139

42. Winter CW. *The Sleep Solution; Why Your Sleep Is Broken and How to Fix It.* New York: Random House; 2017.

43. Grønli J, Byrkjedal IK, Bjorvatn B, Nødtvedt Ø, Hamre B, Pallesen S. Reading from an iPad or from a book in bed: the impact on human sleep. A randomized controlled crossover trial. *Sleep Med.* 2016;21:86-92. doi:10.1016/j.sleep.2016.02.006

44. Shin M, Halaki M, Swan P, Ireland AH, Chow CM. The effects of fabric for sleepwear and bedding on sleep at ambient temperatures of 17°C and 22°C. *Nat Sci Sleep.* 2016;8:121-131. doi:10.2147/NSS.S100271

45. Wolpe J. *The Practice of Behavior Therapy.* 2. ed., 2. print. New York: Pergamon Pr; 1973.

46. Jacobs GD. *Say Good Night to Insomnia.* Updated ed. New York: Henry Holt; 2009.

47. Glovinsky P, Spielman A. *The Insomnia Answer: A Personalized Program for Identifying and Overcoming the Three Types of Insomnia.* New York: Perigee Book; 2006.

48. Reid LD. Endogenous opioid peptides and regulation of drinking and feeding. *Am J Clin Nutr.* 1985;42(5 Suppl):1099-1132. doi:10.1093/ajcn/42.5.1099

49. Barlow DH, Durand VM, Hofmann SG. *Abnormal Psychology: An Integrative Approach.*; 2018.

50. Nolen-Hoeksema S. *Women Conquering Depression: How to Gain Control of Eating, Drinking, and Overthinking and Embrace a Healthier Life*.; 2010. https://www.overdrive.com/search?q=1A4F11B7-25E0-4320-9FDF-B4A2A005234F. Accessed November 2, 2018.

51. Nolen-Hoeksema S. *Women Who Think Too Much: How to Break Free of Overthinking and Reclaim Your Life*. New York: St. Martin's Griffin; 2004.

Appendix

Here are some charts that will be useful in keeping track of your progress toward managing your insomnia. Recording your activities provides feedback and, therefore, strengthens the activities.

In addition to using the charts, you might also keep a dairy of your thoughts as you attempt the mission of overcoming chronic insomnia. Doing such activity often clarifies thinking.

Each morning of your 6-week schedule to consolidate habits that will manage insomnia, place a letter in the appropriate box. There are 10 questions a day and that should not take a lot of time. Just write in the book.

	Week 1							
Day		S	M	T	W	T	F	S
Today I woke up with an alarm?								
a. No								
b. Yes								
Today I woke up feeling:								
a. Well-rested								
b. Somewhat rested								
c. Not rested, tired								
How long did it take to fall asleep?								
a. Less than usual or an OK time								
b. More than usual								
I took a nap yesterday:								
a. No								
b. Yes								
I woke up during the night:								
a. No								
b. Yes								
I used my cued relaxation skills when needed:								
a. Often								
b. Sometimes								
c. Not at all								
I responded to my three reminders:								
a. Always								
b. Sometimes								
c. Not at all								
I used drugs to get to sleep:								
a. No								
b. Yes								
I did things to modify the bedroom/place where I sleep:								
a. Yes								
b. No								
I practiced mindfullness skills:								
a. Yes								
b. No								

	Week 2							
Day		S	M	T	W	T	F	S
Today I woke up with an alarm?								
a. No								
b. Yes								
Today I woke up feeling:								
a. Well-rested								
b. Somewhat rested								
c. Not rested, tired								
How long did it take to fall asleep?								
a. Less than usual or an OK time								
b. More than usual								
I took a nap yesterday:								
a. No								
b. Yes								
I woke up during the night:								
a. No								
b. Yes								
I used my cued relaxation skills when needed:								
a. Often								
b. Sometimes								
c. Not at all								
I responded to my three reminders:								
a. Always								
b. Sometimes								
c. Not at all								
I used drugs to get to sleep:								
a. No								
b. Yes								
I did things to modify the bedroom/place where I sleep:								
a. Yes								
b. No								
I practiced mindfullness skills:								
a. Yes								
b. No								

	Week 3							
	Day	S	M	T	W	T	F	S
Today I woke up with an alarm?								
a. No								
b. Yes								
Today I woke up feeling:								
a. Well-rested								
b. Somewhat rested								
c. Not rested, tired								
How long did it take to fall asleep?								
a. Less than usual or an OK time								
b. More than usual								
I took a nap yesterday:								
a. No								
b. Yes								
I woke up during the night:								
a. No								
b. Yes								
I used my cued relaxation skills when needed:								
a. Often								
b. Sometimes								
c. Not at all								
I responded to my three reminders:								
a. Always								
b. Sometimes								
c. Not at all								
I used drugs to get to sleep:								
a. No								
b. Yes								
I did things to modify the bedroom/place where I sleep:								
a. Yes								
b. No								
I practiced mindfullness skills:								
a. Yes								
b. No								

Week 4

Day	S	M	T	W	T	F	S
Today I woke up with an alarm?							
a. No							
b. Yes							
Today I woke up feeling:							
a. Well-rested							
b. Somewhat rested							
c. Not rested, tired							
How long did it take to fall asleep?							
a. Less than usual or an OK time							
b. More than usual							
I took a nap yesterday:							
a. No							
b. Yes							
I woke up during the night:							
a. No							
b. Yes							
I used my cued relaxation skills when needed:							
a. Often							
b. Sometimes							
c. Not at all							
I responded to my three reminders:							
a. Always							
b. Sometimes							
c. Not at all							
I used drugs to get to sleep:							
a. No							
b. Yes							
I did things to modify the bedroom/place where I sleep:							
a. Yes							
b. No							
I practiced mindfullness skills:							
a. Yes							
b. No							

	Week 5							
Day		S	M	T	W	T	F	S
Today I woke up with an alarm? a. No b. Yes								
Today I woke up feeling: a. Well-rested b. Somewhat rested c. Not rested, tired								
How long did it take to fall asleep? a. Less than usual or an OK time b. More than usual								
I took a nap yesterday: a. No b. Yes								
I woke up during the night: a. No b. Yes								
I used my cued relaxation skills when needed: a. Often b. Sometimes c. Not at all								
I responded to my three reminders: a. Always b. Sometimes c. Not at all								
I used drugs to get to sleep: a. No b. Yes								
I did things to modify the bedroom/place where I sleep: a. Yes b. No								
I practiced mindfullness skills: a. Yes b. No								

	Week 6							
	Day	S	M	T	W	T	F	S
Today I woke up with an alarm? a. No b. Yes								
Today I woke up feeling: a. Well-rested b. Somewhat rested c. Not rested, tired								
How long did it take to fall asleep? a. Less than usual or an OK time b. More than usual								
I took a nap yesterday: a. No b. Yes								
I woke up during the night: a. No b. Yes								
I used my cued relaxation skills when needed: a. Often b. Sometimes c. Not at all								
I responded to my three reminders: a. Always b. Sometimes c. Not at all								
I used drugs to get to sleep: a. No b. Yes								
I did things to modify the bedroom/place where I sleep: a. Yes b. No								
I practiced mindfullness skills: a. Yes b. No								

About the Authors

Professor Larry D. Reid has been teaching at major universities for over 50 years. Among the courses he has taught regularly are Psychopharmacology, Drugs, Society and Behavior and more recently the Psychological Science of Abnormal Behavior. During most of those years he maintained a research laboratory that regularly produced research and involved the publication of books and scientific articles. That research is regularly cited in the scientific literature. He has been recognized for his contributions by being designated as a Fellow of the American Psychological Association, the Association for Psychological Science, and the International Behavioral Neuroscience Society.

Prof. Reid, as of the date of publication of this book, is 82 years old and still is teaching courses. His age almost forces him to think about the looming threat of developing Alzheimer's disease. He has witnessed the ravages of the disease among his contemporaries. Characteristically, he started studying Alzheimer's disease. That study led to a major review on Alzheimer's disease in which he outlined a system for the prevention of the disease. Now, he is almost totally involved with establishing the means of preventing the disease based on the biological nature of the disease; and, the technological advances made in clinical psychology, mainly evidence-based cognitive behavioral interventions. This book is part of that effort.

As Larry began writing this book, he asked a friend, Valerie Lavash, who he knew was brilliant and had good writing skills, to help him make his writing more suitable for the general public. Virtually, every sentence in this book profited from her good work. We worked together to produce this small book and it presents some novel approaches toward the prevention of Alzheimer's disease.

www.ingramcontent.com/pod-product-compliance
Lightning Source LLC
Chambersburg PA
CBHW040216220526
45473CB00001B/8